OXFORD ASSESS

D0262616

Series Editors

Kathy Boursicot
Reader in Medical Education and Deputy Head of the Centre for Medical and Healthcare Education, St George's, University of London

David Sales
Consultant in Medical Assessment

OXFORD ASSESS AND PROGRESS
your prescription for exam success

Written by clinicians and educational experts, these unique guides present complete coverage for your exam revision, with illustrative material and tips to help you suceed in your medical exams.

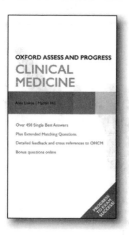

OXFORD ASSESS AND PROGRESS
CLINICAL MEDICINE

Alex Liakos | Hamed Khan

Over 450 Single Best Answers

Plus Extended Matching Questions

Detailed feedback and cross references to OHCM

Bonus questions online

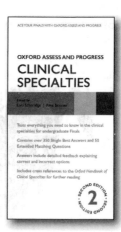

ACE YOUR FINALS WITH OXFORD ASSESS AND PROGRESS

OXFORD ASSESS AND PROGRESS
CLINICAL SPECIALTIES

Edited by
Luci Etheridge | Alex Bonner

Tests everything you need to know in the clinical specialties for undergraduate Finals

Contains over 350 Single Best Answers and 50 Extended Matching Questions

Answers include detailed feedback explaining correct and incorrect options

Includes cross references to the *Oxford Handbook of Clinical Specialties* for further reading

SECOND EDITION · **2** · SECOND EDITION

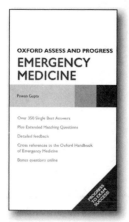

OXFORD ASSESS AND PROGRESS
EMERGENCY MEDICINE

Pawan Gupta

Over 350 Single Best Answers

Plus Extended Matching Questions

Detailed feedback

Cross references to the Oxford Handbook of Emergency Medicine

Bonus questions online

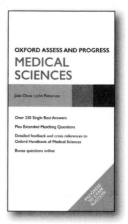

OXFORD ASSESS AND PROGRESS
MEDICAL SCIENCES

Jade Chow | John Patterson

Over 250 Single Best Answers

Plus Extended Matching Questions

Detailed feedback and cross references to Oxford Handbook of Medical Sciences

Bonus questions online

www.oup.com

OXFORD ASSESS AND PROGRESS

Situational
Judgement Test

Harveer Dev
Cambridge University Hospital NHS Foundation Trust

David Metcalfe
St George's Healthcare NHS Trust

OXFORD
UNIVERSITY PRESS

OXFORD
UNIVERSITY PRESS

Great Clarendon Street, Oxford, OX2 6DP,
United Kingdom

Oxford University Press is a department of the University of Oxford.
It furthers the University's objective of excellence in research, scholarship,
and education by publishing worldwide. Oxford is a registered trade mark of
Oxford University Press in the UK and in certain other countries

© Oxford University Press, 2012

The moral rights of the authors have been asserted

First Edition published 2012

Impression: 1

British Library Cataloguing in Publication Data
Data available

Library of Congress Cataloging in Publication Data
Library of Congress Control Number: 2012944658

ISBN 978–0–19–966036–0

Printed in Italy by
L.E.G.O S.p.A. — Lavis TN

Foreword

Being a doctor is a huge privilege: we touch and change lives and enjoy unparalleled levels of public trust. But the high reputation enjoyed by the medical profession depends on all who practise medicine behaving in a way that continues to command confidence and respect. A great deal of what we do depends on knowledge and skills, and we all keep learning new facts or embracing new ideas throughout our careers. But there is another and equally important aspect of being a doctor and that is about knowing our limitations. Really good doctors will know the limit of what they know and what they can do. No one—most of all the patient you're seeing at that moment—will thank you for doing something that you're simply not able to do. Whether it's thinking that you remember the dose of a drug but not checking, or soldiering on because you think it's a sign of weakness to ask for help, or advising someone about the risks of a procedure you've never done, or a myriad of other pitfalls, knowing the limits of your own abilities is one of a doctor's most important qualities.

The General Medical Council has been guiding doctors in the area of professionalism for over 150 years. The world has changed a lot over that time, but some of the qualities that define the physician are timeless and have endured. This book guides you through various scenarios where your professionalism could be tested and helpfully references some of our guidance. The message is simple but fundamentally important: saying that you don't know, but will find someone who does, is a sign of professional maturity.

Professor Sir Peter Rubin
Chair, General Medical Council

Series Editor Preface

The *Oxford Assess and Progress Series* started as a groundbreaking development in the extensive area of self-assessment texts available for medical studies. The majority of volumes are linked to the *Oxford Handbook* series, with specially commissioned modern format questions constructed to test the problem-solving skills used by practising clinicians in order to deliver high quality and safe patient care by recognizing, understanding, and treating common problems as well as recognizing less likely, but potentially catastrophic, conditions.

With the increasing emphasis on the professionalism of doctors, and the requirement to test and demonstrate professional values and behaviour, a new format of questions has been developed and introduced into selection procedures for a number of postgraduate education and training circumstances. These questions are known collectively as a Situational Judgement Test (SJT), which is designed to test certain attributes deemed to be desirable in practising medical professionals, encompassing the values, attitudes, and behaviours expected of new doctors as set out in the General Medical Council's documents *Good Medical Practice* (2012) and *Tomorrow's Doctors* (2009).

This particular volume is special as it is written for this new question format, but in keeping with the rest of the series it has a number of unique features and is designed as much as a formative learning resource as a self-assessment one. The current position of the SJT within the selection to the Foundation Programme in the UK is explained in detail, with advice on how to approach this new set of tests.

The test items place the candidate in professionally challenging situations, and a number of possible reactions are offered. Attention has been paid to explaining learning points and constructive feedback on each question, using clear fact- or evidence-based explanations as to why the 'correct' response is the most appropriate and why the other responses are less appropriate. This is especially important as SJTs require consideration of the most appropriate responses to a given professional dilemma, where no single answer is completely correct or incorrect.

As the use of SJTs is likely to expand into more contexts where doctors' professionalism, values, and attitudes will be formally tested, this volume is a leading-edge introduction on how to prepare for the future of such testing.

Kathy Boursicot
2012

Author Preface

With finals on the horizon, you might be tempted to coast through the Situational Judgement Test (SJT). The Foundation Programme is *generic* as all trainees develop the same core skills and competencies, and you might be told that your choice of FY1/FY2 rotations 'doesn't really matter'.

The truth is that your clinical rotations might easily shape the rest of your career. It's unsurprising that most doctors settle in the area to which they are allocated for their first job. But your rotations are also important for progressing to the next stage of your chosen specialty. Although specific clinical experience is never mandatory, it is easier to argue convincingly that you want to work in a specialty if you have relevant audit projects, contacts, and experience. The best way to develop a specialty-specific portfolio is to secure your first choice rotation. If you have strong feelings about where you want to work or your future specialty, you need to maximize your SJT score.

You might also hear that you 'can't study' for the SJT. We have sat many exams between us and have yet to come across one which can't be beaten with hard work and adequate preparation.

This book will help you become familiar with the style and content of SJT questions. Practice questions and familiarity with professional guidance are vital to maximizing your SJT score.

Best of luck with the SJT and securing your first choice rotation!

Harveer Dev
David Metcalfe

Acknowledgements

It would not have been possible to produce this book without the help of many individuals and their institutions. In particular:

All the reviewers (pp. xiv–xv) who helped to produce thought-provoking questions and carefully considered explanations.

The invaluable principles laid out by the General Medical Council (p. 18) on which our answers are based. In particular, we must thank Professor Sir Peter Rubin for contributing the Preface.

Our editorial team at Oxford University Press, specifically Geraldine Jeffers and series editor Katharine Boursicot.

Mina, Jasvinder, and Bobby for their continued support for, and patience with, the editors.

Contents

Series editors

Katharine Boursicot is a Reader in Medical Education and Deputy Head of the Centre for Medical and Healthcare Education at St George's, University of London. Previously she was Head of Assessment at Barts and the London NHS Trust, and Associate Dean for Assessment at Cambridge University School of Clinical Medicine. She is consultant on assessment to several UK medical schools, medical Royal Colleges, and international institutions, as well as a consultant on the General Medical Council Professional and Linguistic Assessments Board Part 2 Panel and Fitness to Practise clinical skills testing.

David Sales is a general practitioner by training who has been involved in medical assessment for over 20 years, having previously been convenor of the MRCGP knowledge test. He has run item-writing workshops for a number of undergraduate medical schools and medical Royal Colleges, and internationally. He currently chairs the Professional and Linguistic Assessments Board Part 1 panel for the General Medical Council, and is their consultant on Fitness to Practise knowledge testing.

About the authors

Harveer Dev graduated with a BA(Hons) in Natural Sciences (2008) and an MB BChir (2011) from the University of Cambridge. He has held various pedagogical roles for the University of Cambridge, including as preclinical supervisor for St Edmund's College. He won a number of medical school prizes and undertook an elective in urology at Weill Cornell Medical College (Presbyterian Hospital, New York). Harveer is currently an Academic Foundation Doctor (Urology) at Cambridge University Hospital NHS Foundation Trust.

David Metcalfe graduated with a first-class BSc(Hons) in Biological Sciences with Molecular Genetics (2006) and MB ChB (2010) from the University of Warwick. He won over twenty scholarships and awards at medical school, including the Pridgeon Gold Medal, and was appointed Honorary Research Fellow at St George's Vascular Institute on graduation. David graduated with a first-class qualifying law degree from The Open University (2012) and currently teaches medical ethics and law at University College London.

Reviewers

Laura Barnfield MBChB
Trafford General Hospital,
Manchester, UK

Elizabeth Bird-Lieberman
MA PhD MRCP
University of Cambridge,
Cambridge, UK

Daniel Border BSc(Hons)
MBChB
City Hospital Birmingham,
Birmingham, UK

James Chambers BSc(Hons)
MBChB
Aintree University Hospital,
Liverpool, UK

Dan Cooper BSc(Hons)
MBChB
Royal Liverpool University
Hospital, Liverpool, UK

Susie Cooper MBChB
MRCPCH
Princess Ann Hospital,
Southampton, UK

William Coppola MBCh MA
DRCOG MRCGP
University College London
Medical School London, UK

Harveer Dev BA(Hons)
MBBChir
Addenbrooke's Hospital,
Cambridge, UK

Jon Downing BSc(Hons)
MBChB
Great Western Hospital,
Swindon, UK

Oghenekome Gbinigie
MA(Hons) MBBChir
University College Hospital,
London, UK

John Gomes MBBS PhD
MRCP
London, UK

Ruth Green MEng(Hons) MA
MBBS
St George's Hospital, London, UK

Alison Ho MA MBBS
St Peter's Hospital, Chertsey

Kat Holt BMedSci MBBCh
Medway Maritime Hospital,
Gillingham, UK

Kulvir Hundal MBChB
West Midlands, UK

Tariq Husain BSc(Hons) MA
MRCP FRCA DICM
Northwick Park Hospital,
Harrow, UK

Syed Jafery MBBS
Queen Elizabeth Hospital,
King's Lynn, UK

Reena Johal MBChB
West Midlands, UK

Vasha Kaur MBChB MRCS
London, UK

Jayne Kavanagh BA(Hons) MA
MBChB
University College London,
London, UK

Hugh Mackenzie BSc(Hons)
MRCS
St Mary's Hospital, London, UK

David McKean MA BMBCh
John Radcliffe Hospital,
Oxford, UK

Eleanor Mearing-Smith
BSc(Hons) MRCS
London, UK

Explanation of terms

Most of the terms used in these questions should be familiar, but you should note the following.

Clinical Supervisor
The person directly responsible for your day-to-day clinical practice. This will almost always be one of the consultants leading your team. You should approach them about problems with the team, post, or patients under their care.

Educational Supervisor
The person responsible for your professional development through a number of rotations (e.g. the whole of FY1). They have a more global view of your progress and ensure continuity as you move between posts. You should approach them about career plans, pastoral concerns, and problems with your Clinical Supervisor.

Clinical Director
The senior clinician (usually a consultant) with responsibility for a particular department within a hospital, e.g. the Emergency Department.

Medical Director
A senior doctor (i.e. a consultant) with management responsibilities at a trust level. The Medical Director is generally more senior than the Clinical Directors.

ABG	Arterial Blood Gas
AMTS	Abbreviated Mental Test Score
ALS	Advanced Life Support
ATLS	Advanced Trauma Life Support
CAGE	Concern, Anger, Guilt, Eye opener
CT	Computed Tomography (scan)
DVLA	Driver and Vehicle Licensing Authority
FY1	Foundation Year 1 (doctor)
FY2	Foundation Year 2 (doctor)
GMC	General Medical Council
MDT	Multi-Disciplinary Team
MRI	Magnetic Resonance Imaging
PALS	Patient Advice and Liaison Service
SHO	Senior House Officer
SJT	Situational Judgement Test
TAB	Team Assessment of Behaviour

Section 1

Introduction to the SJT

Chapter 1

Foundation Programme selection

New doctors intending to work in the UK should complete the Foundation Programme. This two-year schedule of rotations ensures core competencies are achieved before doctors enter further training.

Selection to the first foundation year (FY1) is overseen by the UK Foundation Programme Office (UKFPO).

This organization is responsible for allocating final-year medical students to their new foundation schools.

Allocation of posts

Allocation to foundation schools depends on a score achieved by each student. Applicants through UKFPO must rank all foundation schools (Units of Application) during the online application process.

The system begins with the highest-scoring applicant and assigns them their first-choice foundation school. It does the same for the second-highest-scoring applicant and continues in this vein. Once the system reaches an applicant whose first-choice foundation school is 'full', they are assigned their second choice, and so on.

Therefore the key determinants as to whether an applicant is placed in their first choice location are their UKFPO 'score' and the popularity of their chosen foundation school. The ratio of first-choice applicants to places varies every year, but some foundation schools (e.g. Oxford and those in London) are almost always over-subscribed.

Therefore it is important to understand how scores are assigned and maximize your performance on these measures.

Assignment of scores

Until 2012 entry, student preferences were allocated according to two measures.

1. Position within their medical school cohort by quartile. Quartiles were determined locally by each medical school with only general guidance from the UKFPO.
2. Answers provided on an application form which asked about academic achievements but weighted most points towards short essay-type answers.

This system was widely perceived as stressful and unfair by students. Such concerns led to a project called Improving Selection to the Foundation Programme (ISFP). After a wide-ranging review, ISFP has proposed a revised system to distinguish between new doctors. In brief, this will also include two components.

1. Educational Performance Measure (EPM).
2. Situational Judgement Test (SJT).

Educational Performance Measure

The EPM is an attempt at measuring academic performance. It comprises three parts.

1. Medical school performance (34–43).
2. Degrees (0–5).
3. Publications, presentations, and prizes (0–2).

Medical school performance is still determined locally but by deciles to achieve finer discrimination. The assessments counting towards this score and their respective weighting should be (or have been) discussed with your cohort representatives.

The points awarded for various academic achievements are shown in Tables 1.1 and 1.2.

Table 1.1

Qualification	Points
Doctoral degree	5
Masters degree 1st-class honours degree* BDS/BVetMed	4
2.1 honours degree*	3
2.2 honours degree*	2
3rd class, unclassified, or ordinary honours degree*	1
Primary medical qualification	0

*Intercalated degrees which do not extend for the course length are awarded one point less for each honours category.

Table 1.2

Achievement	Points
Prizes First prize national/international educational prize	1
Presentations Oral or poster presentation at a national/international conference	1
Publications Named author on a research paper in a peer-reviewed journal with a PubMed ID (PMID)	1

Be aware that only five points can be awarded for degrees and two for other academic achievements. Therefore a fortunate applicant with a first-class honours BSc(Hons) and PhD will score five points in the degrees category.

Situational Judgement Test

Your EPM score is difficult to influence if you are within a year of applying to the Foundation Programme.

The good news (for most students) is that the EPM is actually the minority component. Officially, the EPM is out of 50 points and SJT scores are similarly recalibrated to a 50-point scale. However, you may recall that the lowest possible EPM score is 34 points (p. 4). This means there are *only 17* possible points between a student in the bottom decile with no academic achievements and the highest achiever with a PhD and a string of publications/presentations/prizes.

Therefore all applicants should seek to maximize their score on the second component—the SJT. Fortunately you are off to a good start by reading this book!

What is the SJT?

Situational judgement tests are commonly used by organizations for personnel selection. They aim to provide realistic but hypothetical scenarios and possible answers which are either selected or ranked by the candidate.

One such test will contribute half, or significantly more than half (see p. 3) the score used by applicants to the UK Foundation Programme.

Mechanics of the SJT

The test will involve a single paper over two hours and twenty minutes in which candidates will answer 70 questions.

In one SJT pilot (p. 16), 96% of candidates finished the test within two hours, which provides some indication about the time pressure. It is important to answer all questions and not simply 'guess' those left at the end. Although the SJT is not negatively marked, random guesses are not allocated points. The scoring software will identify guesses by looking for unusual or sporadic answer patterns.

The SJT will be held locally by individual medical schools under invigilated conditions. Therefore your medical school should be in touch about specific local arrangements.

Each SJT paper will include a selection of questions, each mapped to a specific professional attribute (p. 11). Questions should be evenly distributed between attributes and between scenario type, i.e. 'patient', 'colleague', or 'personal'.

The SJT will include two types of question:

- multiple choice questions (approximately one third)
- ranking questions (approximately two thirds).

Multiple choice questions

These begin with a scenario and provide eight possible answers. Three of these are correct and should be selected. The remaining five are incorrect.

The example in Box 2.1 provides an illustrative medical school scenario. For questions based around foundation programme scenarios, over 100 examples are provided for practice from p. 27 onwards.

Box 2.1

All of your friends have received an email from the medical school allocating a piece of work. You have not received any such correspondence.

Choose the THREE most appropriate actions to take in this situation.

A Ignore the email as it has not been sent to you.

B Write a complaint to the administrator as she has left you off the mailing list.

C Complete the piece of work and submit it by the deadline.

D Ask the administrator if the email was intended for you as well.

E Keep quiet as this will guarantee you an extension.

F Ask your friends for details to assess whether you should have been included.

G Check whether any other important emails have gone astray.

H Use a friend's work as a basis for your own to save time.

The answer in this case might be D, F, G.

Each correct answer scores four marks, and so the highest score for each question is twelve. It is important to note that if more than three options are chosen, the whole question is awarded zero.

Ranking questions

Ranking questions begin with a scenario and provide five possible answers. You must rank the answers from 'most appropriate' to 'least appropriate'. This is challenging as it may require you to choose between conflicting values. It might also be difficult to determine which of two *inappropriate* actions is the least appropriate.

A medical school example might be along the lines of that shown in Box 2.2.

Box 2.2

You arrive 10 minutes late for a mandatory lecture. As you peer through the doors, you see there are no spaces on the back row and you will have to disturb a number of settled students to find a seat.

Rank in order the following actions in response to this situation (1 = most appropriate; 5 = least appropriate).

A Go to the library and study the lecture material before slipping in for the next session.

B Head into the lecture theatre and move people along the row so that you can get a seat.

C Sign the attendance register and then wait for your friends in the coffee shop.

D Head into the lecture theatre and move a lot of people so you can get to your favourite seat in the middle of a row.

E Go to the coffee shop until the lecture ends and you can slip in for the next session.

The answer in this case might be B, A, E, D, C.

The lecture is mandatory and you should attend, even if this means politely disturbing some of your colleagues (B). Studying the material elsewhere is less ideal as you are supposed to attend the session (A). However, studying the material is preferable to sitting in the coffee shop (E). Sitting in the coffee shop waiting for the next session might in turn be a better option than disturbing many of your colleagues (and potentially the lecture itself) unnecessarily (D). However, the least appropriate option is signing the attendance register when you have not attended the session (C). This is dishonest and casts considerable doubt on your professional probity.

The scoring of such ranking questions is complicated. Each question is marked out of 20 potential points, as illustrated in Fig 2.1.

Figure 2.1

Correct order	Applicant order				
	1	**2**	**3**	**4**	**5**
1	4	3	2	1	0
2	3	4	3	2	1
3	2	3	4	3	2
4	1	2	3	4	3
5	0	1	2	3	4

This system means that a complete answer will always score a minimum of 8/20.

Thus, if you had selected A, D, C, B, E in the above example, your score would be 10/20 as illustrated in Fig. 2.2.

Figure 2.2

Correct order	Applicant order				
	A	**D**	**C**	**B**	**E**
B	4	3	2	1	0
A	3	4	3	2	1
E	2	3	4	3	2
C	1	2	3	4	3
D	0	1	2	3	4

It is important to note that if two options are given the same ranking, both tied options will be awarded zero. Tying options is the only way to score less than eight and so is best avoided unless you are feeling particularly experimental!

What does the SJT test?

The SJT was developed to test nine professional attributes identified from a detailed analysis of the FY1 role. These attributes are as follows.

1. Commitment to professionalism
2. Coping with pressure
3. Effective communication
4. Learning and professional development
5. Organization and planning
6. Patient focus
7. Problem-solving and decision-making
8. Self-awareness and insight
9. Working effectively as part of a team

However, the SJT recognizes that there is considerable overlap between these attributes and that some cannot be effectively assessed with a written test. As a result, SJT questions focus on the five attributes highlighted in bold.

It is worth considering what the SJT requires of candidates according to each key attribute.

Commitment to professionalism

Candidates must be honest, trustworthy, reliable, and aware of ethical issues (e.g. confidentiality). They should challenge behaviour that is unacceptable or risks patient safety. Candidates should take appropriate responsibility for their own actions and omissions.

Coping with pressure

Candidates must be resilient and remain calm under pressure. Judgement should not be affected by pressure and candidates should develop appropriate coping strategies.

Effective communication

Candidates should communicate (verbally and in writing) concisely and clearly. They should be able to vary their communication style appropriately and to negotiate, and be willing to engage others in open dialogue.

Patient focus

Candidates should always show respect to patients. They should adopt a collaborative approach to decision-making with patients as well as maintaining courtesy, empathy, and compassion.

Working effectively as part of a team

Candidates should be able to work in partnership while respecting different views. They should share tasks fairly and ask advice from others when necessary.

Should not *would* questions

Despite appearances, the SJT is a *knowledge-based* examination. It is important to remember throughout that questions ask what you *should* do rather than what you *would* do in any given situation. Therefore it is a test of whether you know the 'correct' action and not whether you would act correctly if working as a doctor.

For example, a question might introduce you as an FY1 doctor on a busy ward. You are told to examine an elderly patient of the opposite sex and all the nurses are occupied elsewhere. You might have seen doctors examine patients under these circumstances without a chaperone. You might even think that this would be your approach in real life. However, you know on some level that a better solution is to insist on (or at least to offer) the presence of a chaperone. Therefore this option is likely to rank above continuing to examine the patient.

Does it work?

Improving Selection to the Foundation Programme (ISFP) undertook a wide-ranging review of options for allocating new doctors to FY1 posts. It selected the SJT.

Whether the SJT works or not depends on whether it can accurately predict 'good' doctors. There is no real consensus about how to measure the effectiveness of foundation doctors, and so the SJT question is unlikely to ever be resolved to everyone's satisfaction. However, variations on the SJT have been used in selection to some specialties (e.g. GP and public health training). They are also used by many firms in the commercial sector.

The SJT pilots suggested a high degree of internal reliability ($\alpha = 0.79$–0.85). It was also shown that SJT performance is positively correlated with extraversion, openness, and achievement.

Advantages of the SJT over the previously used 'white space'questions (p. 3) include the following.

- Invigilated conditions so that no one can seek external help with answers.
- Less reliance on creative writing skills.
- Questions directly address prioritization, team-working, and professionalism—all of which are important qualities for new doctors.
- Evidence from other sectors suggests that situational judgement questions can effectively predict job performance.

Although students are unlikely to relish sitting another high-stakes examination in their final year, earlier selection methods were perceived as both burdensome and unfair. It is impossible to please everyone and you are most likely to approve of this method in retrospect if your score is high enough.

How are SJT questions created?

The SJT questions were created following the professional attributes (p. 11) identified from the FY1 job analysis.

Question writing

Questions were written by volunteers at a series of dedicated workshops. The volunteers were not all doctors but had to be familiar with the FY1 role and have worked with junior doctors within the previous two years.

The ISFP Project Group employed 89 people to write SJT questions, of whom 69 (77.5%) were senior doctors, two (2.2%) were lay representatives, and the remainder were undeclared. In terms of background, 59 (66.3%) were from a range of acute specialties and 12 (13.5%) from community specialties.

Two-part review process

This team created a bank of 453 possible questions. These were scrutinized by a team of psychologists who accepted 360 questions as passing this initial stage.

A select few writers were asked to moderate all questions to ensure that scenarios were realistic and the terminology was in use across the UK. This group eliminated additional questions, leaving a total of 306.

Foundation doctor focus groups

A series of focus groups were then held with foundation doctors who scrutinized the test instructions and up to 20 questions each. They proposed a number of amendments and whittled down the total question bank to 275 items.

Concordance panel

Once a question bank was established, it was trialled using a panel of subject 'experts', i.e. people with similar qualifications to the question writers.

Questions survived this process if they achieved a satisfactory level of concordance, i.e. enough experts independently arrived at the same answer under test conditions. A total of 200 questions went forward to be used in the SJT pilots.

SJT pilots

The SJT model underwent two pilots. The second and larger of these took place in 13 UK medical schools, involving 639 final-year students. Students reported that the content seemed relevant to the Foundation Programme (85% agreed) and that the questions were fair (73.3%).

Why does this matter?

The reasons for understanding how questions are created are to appreciate the following.

- A lot of thought has gone into every question. There should be no ambiguities (unless intended) or 'tricks'.
- They are written (largely) by senior doctors who are presumably interested in medical training and development. This is the perspective informing both questions and answers.
- The question pool is relatively small as the number of possible scenarios is limited. This makes it easier to prepare for the SJT (p. 17) than might otherwise be imagined.

How can you prepare?

The Improving Selection to the Foundation Programme (ISFP) project does not believe that it is possible to be 'coached' through the SJT. This is generally true. Knowing the 'right thing to do' in any given situation is a matter of internalized values and intuition.

However, no one seriously accepts that candidates are born with a fixed level of situational judgement. This is clearly something which develops over time and therefore can change.

In addition, the SJT does not set out to test *your* values but whether you *understand* the values and attitudes expected of a FY1 doctor. This is why you are instructed to answer questions as you 'should', not as you 'would'.

The principles on which foundation doctors should base their behaviour are learned and internalized throughout medical school. However, knowledge of these principles can clearly be learned in the same way as any other part of the medical school curriculum.

Is the SJT worth preparing for?

Most final-year medical students are satisfied with the FY1 posts to which they are allocated. For 2012 entry, 92% were appointed to their top five foundation schools. Those who are not initially pleased often look back in retrospect and are satisfied with their allocations. Your score on the SJT is unlikely to make or break your career.

However, the same can be said of medical school finals. You will almost certainly pass finals—upwards of 95% of final-year students do so—and your ultimate career destination is unlikely to hinge on your cumulative examination score. But this is *not* a reason to go into finals unprepared.

The truth is that every point on the SJT, as in finals, could mean the difference between your chosen outcome and something different. A point lost on the SJT could result in your leaving your first-choice foundation school and moving across the country for work, or not having a high enough score to capture your chosen specialty as a Foundation Programme rotation.

Increasing competition for FY1 posts means that not everyone can be appointed. In 2012, there were 81 more applications than available posts. Although this is a small number in a pool of 7000+ applicants, it should be taken seriously.

Although you may be told otherwise, the SJT *is* a high-stakes examination. If other students choose not to maximize their score ('because you can't prepare for this type of test…'), this is your opportunity to step ahead of the curve. If your colleagues are preparing, you need to redouble your efforts.

How can you prepare?

The values, attitudes, and behaviours expected of new doctors are help-fully recorded in a set of publicly available documents.

SJT question writers, whether explicitly or otherwise, will have inter-nalized these principles over many years and used them to inform their answers. When doubt arose about the correct answer, these principles would have been definitive.

At some point in your preparation, you should read the following four documents.

- General Medical Council (www.gmc-uk.org):
  - *Good Medical Practice* (2012)
  - *Tomorrow's Doctors* (2009), particularly 'Outcomes 3—the Doctor as a Professional'.
- UK Foundation Programme (www.foundationprogramme.nhs.uk):
  - *Person Specification for Recruitment to the Foundation Programme*
  - *Foundation Programme Curriculum*.

As you read, you may feel that each statement is 'obvious'. This is because you began internalizing their contents years ago. Try to concen-trate, though, as their balance of priorities may be subtly different and shift your understanding, whether or not you realize this at the time.

If you have time, the GMC produces a vast amount of guidance, all of which could aid your approach to the SJT. The following documents, avail-able electronically from the GMC website, might be useful:

- *0–18 Years: Guidance for All Doctors* (2007)
- *Accountability in Multi-Disciplinary and Multi-Agency Mental Health Teams* (2005)
- *Confidentiality* (2009)
- *Consent: Patients and Doctors Making Decisions Together* (2008)
- *Good Practice in Prescribing Medicines* (2008)
- *Good Practice in Research and Consent to Research* (2010)
- *Leadership and Management for All Doctors* (2012)
- *Maintaining Boundaries* (2006)
- *Personal Beliefs and Medical Practice* (2008)
- *Raising and Acting on Concerns About Patient Safety* (2012)
- *Reporting Convictions: Reporting Criminal and Regulatory Proceedings Within and Outside the UK* (2008)
- *The Trainee Doctor* (2011)
- *Treatment and Care Towards the End of Life* (2010)

What about practice questions?

This is a book of practice questions. There are three ways that complet-ing SJT-type questions that will help you to maximize your score.

- Completing questions is a more active process than reading policy documents. Choosing the correct answer requires concentration.

This will help you to internalize the values and attitudes described previously (p. 17). Seeing our explanations will make you think harder about the issues, particularly if you disagree with our answers!

- You will begin to intuitively spot phrases which indicate the appropriateness of each answer.

There are only 275 items in the official SJT question bank. This is because there are a limited number of realistic scenarios which can be imagined as happening to FY1 doctors. This book presents over 200 such questions and there is likely to be considerable overlap. Complete all 200 questions and you will have thought (reasonably) hard about every scenario that you will encounter in the SJT.

Tips for the SJT

1. Put yourself in the position of a new FY1 doctor when answering each question. But remember that they are asking what you *should* do, not what you *would* do.
2. You should be a paragon of virtue when answering all questions. Remember always that you are unfailingly honest, respectful, open, and fair to colleagues, patients, and relatives alike. It is difficult to imagine scenarios with answers which would require you to be otherwise.
3. If a question involves patient safety (e.g. critically unwell patient, drug error, etc), your priority must *always* be making the patient safe.
4. The well-being of your patient is your first priority. Other considerations (e.g. relatives, targets, fear of being told off, going home on time) are always secondary.
5. 'Seeking senior advice' and 'gathering information' are difficult to criticize and tend to be safe options. Similarly, it is rarely incorrect to document events or complete a formal incident form.
6. Remember your limitations. As an FY1 you should not usually break bad news, consent patients for operations, administer cytotoxic or anaesthetic drugs, or manage critically ill patients without support. 'Call a senior' is the correct answer in these cases.
7. Understand basic concepts of medical law, e.g. when confidentiality can be breached, determining incapacity, consent in children, the doctrine of double effect, detention under the Mental Health Act, etc. You do not need to know specifics (e.g. sections of Acts) but a practical understanding will guide some answers.
8. As an FY1, your Clinical Supervisor is usually a consultant for whom you work during a particular rotation. They are an appropriate source of support for clinical development and problems within the team. Your Educational Supervisor is akin to a Personal Tutor, i.e. responsible for your overall welfare and development throughout the year. They can advise on pastoral issues, professional development, and difficulties with your Clinical Supervisor.
9. Try to complete all questions within the given time-frame as random guesses may be identified by the scoring software and awarded zero (p. 7).

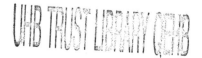

How to use this book

Section 2 of this book is organized into five chapters, each representing a professional attribute to which SJT questions are mapped: commitment to professionalism (Chapter 9, p. 27), coping with pressure (Chapter 10, p. 61), effective communication (Chapter 11, p. 97), patient focus (Chapter 12, p. 131), and working effectively as part of a team (Chapter 13, p. 163). Each section contains 40 questions, split equally between multiple choice and ranking items. The book ends with Section 3 which contains an abbreviated practice test (Chapter 14, p. 199) that uses a mix of different questions.

You will notice throughout the book that most questions cover multiple domains. This is true for those in the SJT as well. It is easy to imagine scenarios which test all five domains with very little effort; for example, a senior nurse pressures you to do something to the detriment of a patient. Do not become distracted by trying to guess which domain(s) are being tested.

Although the SJT requires knowledge (p. 18), the answers to questions cannot be learned by rote. This is what the test creators mean when they say candidates cannot be 'coached' to score highly. The benefit in working through these examples is to think about the issues they raise. For this reason, the 'wrong' answers are at least as valuable as those that are 'correct'.

When practising questions in other subjects (e.g. anatomy), most students read the question, choose an answer, and then check that they picked correctly. The best approach to this book is to read a scenario and then consciously think about which details make (C) a better choice than (D), or vice versa. Only when you have done this should you check our answer and explanation.

SJT questions go through a commendably thorough process of assessment and evaluation (p. 15). The answers are determined by a consensus panel of 'experts', most of whom are senior doctors.

Our own questions have been through an abbreviated review process using the contributors listed on pp. xiv–xv. This group broadly reflect those used by the SJT team to validate their items, i.e. members include Clinical Supervisors, doctors with recent experience of the Foundation Programme, and others working closely with FY1s (e.g. senior nurses). Despite our checks, you may disagree with some answers. Hopefully the accompanying explanation will convince you otherwise, but there is certainly room for disagreement. As long as you have carefully considered the issues raised by each question, it has fulfilled its purpose.

As you work through the questions, you will notice that certain themes arise again and again. This is because, although the facts of each scenario are infinite, only a small number of values and attitudes are expected of FY1 doctors. This explains why there are only 275 items in the SJT question bank (p. 15). Once questions feel repetitive, you have probably begun to identify the most appropriate answers intuitively. You might then be persuaded to try the practice test (p. 199).

Section 2

Questions

Commitment to professionalism

Introduction

Questions within this section will test your probity by exploring responses to scenarios which might require you to challenge unacceptable behaviour, maintain confidentiality, and, as always, prioritize patient safety. You need to demonstrate a commitment to achieving your various clinical responsibilities, as well as a desire for continued learning and a commitment to helping the development of others. These scenarios test your honesty towards patients and colleagues, and a willingness to admit mistakes.

The minimum professional standards required of all doctors are found in the corpus of documents published by the GMC (p. 18).

- These questions will set up circumstances designed to distract you from acting professionally. Do not be fooled.
- Always be willing to challenge unprofessional behaviour exhibited by colleagues, but do so in an appropriate manner.
- Be open about your mistakes to both colleagues and patients. Never be tempted to 'cover up' errors whether they are your own or a colleague's.

QUESTIONS

1. A junior colleague on your team always takes his copy of the patient list home as there is no confidential waste bin on the ward. He says this also helps him prepare for the following day as he can memorize details in time for the consultant ward round.

Rank in order the following actions in response to this situation (1 = Most appropriate; 5 = Least appropriate)

A Tell him this is unfair as he is 'getting ahead' and making you look disorganized by knowing patient details before the ward round.

B Ask Matron or a Senior Sister about obtaining a confidential waste bin.

C Let your colleague know that he should not be taking a patient list home each day.

D Speak to the consultant about your colleague's behaviour.

E Take your own list home so that you can be as familiar with the patients as your colleague.

2. A patient on your ward is HIV positive. He is from a minority community which he feels might react negatively if they knew of his diagnosis. As a result, he is very anxious that no one (including his close family) should be told.

Rank in order the following actions in response to this situation (1 = Most appropriate; 5 = Least appropriate)

A Eliminate all mention of HIV from his notes.

B Amend your patient list so this detail is missing or obscured (e.g. 'retroviral illness').

C Ensure the safety of other doctors and phlebotomists by writing 'HIV+' on blood requests.

D Tell the patient that he should talk to his family as you cannot guarantee complete confidentiality.

E Continue as you would for any other patient under your care.

3. You are sitting in the pub opposite your hospital after work. A group of doctors and nurses from another department are talking loudly and joking about patients on their ward. These patients could easily be identified from the conversations you are overhearing.

*Rank in order the following actions in response to this situation
(1 = Most appropriate; 5 = Least appropriate)*

A Speak to the person who is speaking loudest so he is aware that his behaviour is inappropriate.

B Call hospital security and ask them to intervene.

C Challenge the whole group so that they are aware that their behaviour is inappropriate.

D Contact a manager in their department the following day to alert them to this breach.

E Ignore the situation as they should know better and you do not want to cause a scene.

4. As you arrive on the ward one morning, you hear a nurse in a side room shouting at a patient. The tone and language used are unpleasant. You know that the patient is elderly and has severe dementia.

*Rank in order the following actions in response to this situation
(1 = Most appropriate; 5 = Least appropriate)*

A Knock on the door and ask to speak with the nurse.

B Discuss the issue with a senior nurse (e.g. Matron) in the first instance as soon as they arrive.

C Make preliminary enquiries from other staff working that night to ask if they have noticed inappropriate behaviour.

D Use body language to show your disapproval but do nothing formally as patient safety is not at risk.

E Contact the Care Quality Commission anonymously to avoid raising the issue with employees of your Trust.

5. You begin induction at your new Trust and are asked to sign a number of agreements. One of these is an agreement never to raise concerns with bodies outside of your employing organization. This is a condition of taking up your post.

Rank in order the following actions in response to this situation
(1 = Most appropriate; 5 = Least appropriate)

A Sign the form and begin work as instructed.

B Throw the form away and hope that no one notices that it was not returned.

C Explain that you cannot sign as this prohibits you raising concerns appropriately about patient welfare.

D Sign the form but resolve to raise concerns about patient safety in whatever way is necessary to ensure their resolution.

E Contact your medical defence organization or the GMC for advice if in doubt.

6. You are on call and asked to prescribe amoxicillin for a patient complaining of pain on urination. The nurse has tested his urine which shows leucocytes and nitrites characteristic of a urinary tract infection. Amoxicillin is the suggested treatment according to local protocol.

Rank in order the following actions in response to this situation
(1 = Most appropriate; 5 = Least appropriate)

A Thank the nurse for being proactive and prescribe amoxicillin.

B Prescribe trimethoprim as this is the antibiotic of choice according to your recollections from medical school.

C Review the patient yourself and then prescribe if necessary.

D Reprimand the nurse for testing the urine without instruction.

E Explain that you will only prescribe antibiotics if the patient becomes confused or haemodynamically compromised.

7. You feel under-staffed and under-supported when on call. Together with an FY2 doctor, you are responsible for all new medical admissions and the welfare of around 300 ward patients. Attempts to raise your concern with managers, your Educational Supervisor, and the Clinical Director have been unsuccessful.

Rank in order the following actions in response to this situation (1 = Most appropriate; 5 = Least appropriate)

A Contact the Medical Director and, if necessary, the Trust Chairman

B Document each stage of your complaint carefully.

C Contact a documentary programme and offer to carry a hidden camera to capture specific problems.

D Write an article for your local newspaper raising concerns about patient safety.

E Carry on and do your best whenever you are on call.

8. Your consultant knows that you are interested in his specialty and suggests that you attend a one-day course in another city the following week. You recognize that this would be a good opportunity for professional development. Unfortunately you have no remaining annual leave days and are not entitled to study leave. The rota administrator says that you cannot have time off to attend.

Rank in order the following actions in response to this situation (1 = Most appropriate; 5 = Least appropriate)

A Ask your SHO if she will look after the ward in your absence and go if she agrees.

B Speak to your Educational Supervisor and, with their support, ask the service manager for special permission.

C Accept that you cannot attend the course.

D Add up the number of days that you worked late the week before and attend the course as you are owed enough hours in lieu.

E Attend the course as you already have your consultant's permission.

9. An elderly patient's daughter tells you that she is concerned about the ward care of her mother. She is thinking about writing a formal complaint, and asks you if she is over-reacting and how best to complain.

Rank in order the following actions in response to this situation
(1 = Most appropriate; 5 = Least appropriate)

A Tell her that you will look into things but that a formal complaint will not help.

B Suggest that she drops into the Patient Advice and Liaison Service (PALS) to see what they can offer.

C Explore her concerns and try to clear up any misunderstandings.

D Let your consultant and/or the Ward Sister know that the daughter is dissatisfied and that a formal complaint might follow.

E Tell the daughter that the ward nurses are particularly bad and that she should complain.

10. You are reviewing the drug chart of Tim, a young male patient with a previous anaphylactic reaction to penicillin. Your registrar has prescribed Tazocin which you know contains a penicillin antibiotic. The patient has not yet received his first dose.

Rank in order the following actions in response to this situation
(1 = Most appropriate; 5 = Least appropriate)

A Strike out the prescription and let the nurse know that it should not be administered.

B Complete a clinical incident form.

C Speak with the registrar to alert him/her to this error.

D Ensure that the allergy is recorded clearly on the drug chart and in the patient's notes.

E Amend the prescription, but do not cause a fuss as no harm was done.

11. You are concerned that patients on your ward are rarely seen by a senior doctor. They are reviewed weekly by a registrar but almost never by consultants, who seem to be working at a private hospital most of the time. You are uncertain whether to raise the issue or how you would do this as both your Clinical and Educational Supervisors are consultants within this department. You are deciding whom to contact for advice.

Choose the THREE most appropriate actions to take in this situation

A The consultant who seems most absent from the department and is known to have the biggest private practice.

B Your partner.

C Your medical defence organization.

D A friend from school whose judgement you trust and is now a solicitor.

E An Employer Liaison Officer at the General Medical Council.

F A consultant in another department who is known for his fierce opposition to private practice.

G An SHO who spends his weekends at the private hospital assisting in theatre.

H A senior non-clinical colleague (e.g. a manager).

12. A medical student approaches you for advice. He is very concerned that your consultant has asked students to perform rectal examinations on patients under general anaesthesia without consent. You doubt that this is possible and suspect consent must have been obtained beforehand.

Choose the THREE most appropriate actions to take in this situation

A Warn the student not to say anything as he will upset the consultant and/or make him angry.

B Explain that the consultant is very professional and that consent might have been obtained beforehand.

C Explain that consent was probably obtained beforehand and that the student should do as instructed in theatre.

D Advise the student to ask the consultant if there is doubt about the consent process.

E Warn the student not to say anything as he needs the consultant's support to pass the rotation.

F Tell the student that specific consent for him is not required for some procedures (e.g. rectal cancer resection).

G Advise the student to mention this on the anonymous feedback after the rotation ends.

H Suggest that the student speaks to an appropriate person at his medical school if in doubt.

13. You are the surgical FY1 and hear that an unconscious patient in A&E resuscitation has a ruptured abdominal aortic aneurysm (AAA). Your SHO tells you to feel the patient's abdomen as this is a rare opportunity to feel the expansile mass you read about in textbooks. You have never felt a ruptured AAA before.

Choose the THREE most appropriate actions to take in this situation

A Decline to examine the patient as you do not have consent.

B Make a note to read about abdominal aortic aneurysms as this is not something you have encountered properly before

C Find your medical students so that they can examine the patient as well.

D Examine the patient as this is a valuable learning opportunity.

E Introduce yourself to the most senior doctor present and ask if you can examine the patient.

F Tell your SHO that you are busy on the ward and will go later if you have time.

G Call the patient's next of kin at home to ask if you can examine her father.

H Tell your SHO that you will only examine the patient if he completes a work-based assessment for your e-portfolio.

14. You are a medical FY1 seeing a new patient in A&E. This could be an opportunity to ask your senior to complete a work-based assessment for your e-portfolio. The assessment requires a senior doctor to observe you examining a patient and then complete an electronic form. You ask the medical registrar who says she is too busy to help. Your SHO overhears and offers to complete the assessment without seeing you examine the patient.

Choose the THREE most appropriate actions to take in this situation

A Thank the registrar and ask if you could present the case to her later for your own experience.

B Tell the registrar that you need senior feedback if you are to develop as a doctor.

C Thank the SHO and forward him an electronic form to complete.

D Ask the SHO if he will complete two work-based assessments at the same time.

E Ask the SHO to watch you examine the patient and then complete an assessment.

F Examine the patient as formally as possible, even though you are not being assessed.

G Examine the patient a few hours later when someone might be available to assess you.

H Tell your Educational Supervisor how difficult it is to get senior colleagues to complete formal assessments

15. You are an FY1 doctor required to attend mandatory teaching on Tuesday afternoon. This is also the time that your consultant holds his only ward round of the week. Your registrar is unimpressed that you want to 'slip off' when you are needed to update the consultant on each patient's progress. He suggests that you sign the attendance register then return to the ward round.

Choose the THREE most appropriate actions to take in this situation

A Explain that teaching is mandatory and you are required to attend.

B Sign the attendance register so that your progression through FY1 is not obstructed, and then attend the ward round.

C Agree that your presence on the ward round is necessary and that you will miss teaching.

D Speak with your consultant and explain that your commitments are conflicting.

E Offer to update your registrar about each patient so that he can facilitate the ward round in your place.

F Explain that teaching is mandatory and then go to the doctors' mess for a long break.

G Attend the ward round but read up on the teaching you missed afterwards.

H Send a text message asking an FY1 colleague to sign you in to teaching.

16. Your consultant has two third-year medical students and asks you to teach them for a day. You are a new FY1 who is not yet confident with the role and feel that you are too busy to look after students.

Choose the THREE most appropriate actions to take in this situation

A Tell your consultant that you are far too busy to look after students.

B Wait until your consultant has left, and then sign the students' attendance forms and send them away.

C Wait until your consultant has left and then tell the students that you are too busy.

D Give your bleep to a colleague and deliver a 60 minute tutorial on a topic of your choice.

E Ask the students about their experience so far, their time on the firm, and what they hope to gain.

F Give the students clear tasks which match their learning objectives and help you if possible.

G Ask the students to spend the morning completing discharge summaries which you will check and sign afterwards.

H Ask the students questions about topics with which you are particularly comfortable.

17. You are coming to the end of FY1 and are being shadowed by the final-year medical student intended to replace you. You are very concerned about his attitude towards other healthcare professionals and have received negative feedback from the nursing staff. After five weeks, he asks you to complete a feedback form for his medical school.

Choose the THREE most appropriate actions to take in this situation

A Tell the student throughout the placement that he should adjust his attitude.

B Wait until the end of the placement and then meet somewhere privately to discuss your concerns.

C Tell the student about your concerns but mark all performance domains as 'satisfactory'.

D Let your Clinical Supervisor know that the incoming FY1 has a bad attitude.

E Indicate your concerns on the feedback form with specific examples.

F Give the student an opportunity to discuss your feedback.

G Write to the medical school dean suggesting that formal action be considered.

H Wish the nursing staff 'good luck' working with the incoming FY1.

18. Your Trust has introduced mandatory online prescribing training for specific drugs (e.g. insulin, warfarin, and antibiotics). You are confident working with these drugs and will probably have to complete the training in your own time as your ward commitments are excessive.

Choose the THREE most appropriate actions to take in this situation

A Decline to complete the online modules because there is no time during your working day.

B Complete the online modules quickly, but pick random answers so that you don't have to read the text.

C Ask your Clinical Supervisor or an appropriate manager for protected time in which to complete the modules.

D Complete the modules in your own time without complaint.

E Refuse to complete the modules but satisfy yourself that you can prescribe safely.

F Provide feedback after completing the modules as to whether or not you found them helpful.

G Ask your partner, who is a doctor, to complete the modules for you at home while you are on call.

H Contact the British Medical Association to ask whether you can be forced to complete the modules.

19. A group of five medical students are attached to your firm. You have been spending a lot of time with one of the students and feel that a mutual attraction is developing.

Choose the THREE most appropriate actions to take in this situation

A Try to avoid the student for the rest of the rotation.

B Meet with the student socially so that any romance can develop away from the workplace.

C Try to ensure that your attention is equally distributed between all students on the firm.

D Avoid any romance developing while the student is attached to your firm.

E Tell the student that you are attracted to them but that you should remain professional.

F Ask one of the others whether this particular student is attracted to you.

G Try to avoid unprofessional feelings developing in future.

H Continue with any developing relationship as you are not directly responsible for supervising medical students.

20. You have been looking after Sid, a 90-year-old with endstage heart failure, for a number of months. His condition is worsening. You visit one day and he hands you an envelope containing £500. Although you protest, he insists, saying that it is a 'thank you' and that he 'doesn't need it any more'.

Choose the THREE most appropriate actions to take in this situation

A Tell Sid that the gift is too much and that you will only accept £50.

B Thank Sid for the gift but explain that you are unable to accept.

C Accept the gift and then ask an appropriate person within the Trust whether this is allowed.

D Ask Sid to sign a statement so you are not accused of theft later on.

E Accept the gift but give it to Sid's daughter, who his next of kin, at her next visit.

F Ask him to think carefully about his decision.

G Suggest that he donates the money to your favourite charity instead.

H Ask an appropriate person in the Trust for advice.

21. As the obstetrics and gynaecology FY1, you are called to see a 30-year-old woman who is four hours post partum and is actively bleeding. The patient is a Jehovah 's Witness and you have heard that she would be unwilling to accept blood products. Despite your attempts at fluid resuscitation, the patient continues to bleed. She remains hypotensive and hypoxic, with an Hb of 5.5 and a very low platelet count, although still alert and orientated.

Choose the THREE most appropriate actions to take in this situation

A Transfuse her immediately with red blood cells.

B The woman's decision can be overruled when a child's life is at risk.

C Commence a frank discussion with the patient, highlighting the risks and benefits of the blood transfusion including the possibility of death if she refuses.

D Continue to give intravenous fluids if the patient consents, but do not transfuse any blood products.

E Wait until the patient becomes unconscious before attempting to transfuse blood products.

F Seek the advice of the consultant haemotologist as soon as possible.

G Consider informing the Hospital Liaison Committee for Jehovah's Witnesses.

H Speak to your consultant to initiate the process of overruling the patient's decision with a court order.

22. You are examining a 10-month-old infant in A&E who has been brought in by his parents after an episode of bloody diarrhoea. On examination you find that he has significant scarring secondary to his circumcision. The parents say that the circumcision was performed by an experienced religious leader in accordance with their beliefs.

Rank in order the following actions in response to this situation (1 = Most appropriate; 5 = Least appropriate)

A The scarring does not require treatment on this admission, as it has nothing to do with the presenting complaint.

B Document the findings and discuss the management options with your consultant.

C The examination finding constitutes evidence of genital mutilation, and Child Protection Services should be informed immediately.

D Advise the patient to return to the religious leader for a surgical revision.

E Refer the parents to parenting classes for failing to act in accordance with their child's best interests.

23. You receive your first paycheck as a qualified doctor at the end of a very busy month's work on an understaffed medical ward. You are pleasantly surprised to find that you have received substantial payment for locum shifts, despite having never worked outside your contracted hours. You calculate that the additional hours you have had to work on the medical ward approximate to the additional payment you have received in error.

Rank in order the following actions in response to this situation
(1 = Most appropriate; 5 = Least appropriate)

A Overall, you are receiving the correct amount of payment and are not under any obligation to correct an error made by payroll.

B Write a cheque amounting to 95% of the total additional income that you have been paid for a charity of your choice, retaining a small amount as compensation for your efforts.

C Keep a work diary of the number of hours that you are working.

D Involve your Educational Supervisor, as you should not be working outside your contracted hours.

E Alert payroll to the error so that any additional payment can be docked from your salary.

24. You are preparing your specialty training application for general surgery. You had few opportunities to gain experience in theatre as a foundation doctor. However, you have spoken to many people about surgical careers and watched video recordings of operations. You have booked a Basic Surgical Skills course and read the manual, but have yet to attend it. You are considering what statements you can legitimately make on your application.

Choose the THREE most appropriate actions to take in this situation

A I have enjoyed participating in various operations during my time as a foundation doctor.

B I have enjoyed developing my surgical knowledge through experience as a foundation doctor.

C While I have made every effort to learn about a career in surgery, my Foundation Programme rotations have not allowed time to attend theatre.

D I have managed to gain indirect experience of theatre through watching videos of operations in my spare time.

E I have developed an enthusiasm for the working environment of the operating room through extensive surgical experience.

F I look forward to developing my surgical experience during this surgical specialty training programme.

G I am fully proficient in the Basic Surgical Skills course curriculum.

H My inexperience in the operating room is compensated by a superior command of general medicine.

25. You are completing an orthopaedics audit during one of your FY1 rotations. The consultant surgeon has asked you to review the complication rates for total knee replacements performed at this hospital and compare them with the average across the Trust. Your analysis shows slightly worse postoperative outcomes at this hospital, and the average appears to be significantly skewed by the high complication rates of your consultant.

Rank in order the following actions in response to this situation
(1 = Most appropriate; 5 = Least appropriate)

A Report the consultant surgeon to the Care Quality Commission, as this is an issue of patient safety.

B Ask all the orthopaedic consultants for advice about the data at the following week's departmental meeting.

C Speak with your consultant orthopaedic surgeon privately about the findings.

D Omit your consultant's data, and submit a report without further discussion.

E Obtain further data on preoperative parameters for the cases.

26. After leaving your evening shift as the on-call medical FY1, you walk through the town and come across a group of medical students who have been attached to your ward. They are behaving quite out of character, obviously under the influence of alcohol, and are shouting profanities towards passers-by. The students are eventually confronted by a passing police officer before being asked to move on.

Choose the THREE most appropriate actions to take in this situation

A No further action is necessary, as medical students are not regulated by the same code of practice as doctors.

B Chase the students down the street, and demand that they answer for their actions.

C Inform your Educational Supervisor about what has occurred in the morning.

D Email details of what you observed to the medical school dean.

E Approach the police officer and enquire as to whether further action is needed.

F Confront the medical students about their behaviour the following day.

G Reserve your comments until the end of their medical placement when you are asked to give formal written feedback.

H Withhold any details of the incident from other junior colleagues.

27. During a two-week vacation in Singapore, you became embroiled in an altercation at a bar and were subsequently given a caution by police. You return to work feeling rather upset and ashamed, but determined to put the whole incident behind you.

Rank in order the following actions in response to this situation (1 = Most appropriate; 5 = Least appropriate)

A Try to put the issue behind you.

B Wait until you have settled into your new rotation before raising the issue.

C Inform your Medical Defence Union and seek legal advice.

D Contact the GMC immediately to report the caution.

E Ask your consultant for advice as to how you should proceed.

28. You arrive at work before the consultant ward round and attempt to print the patient list. You are hindered by slow equipment and a broken printer. The ward round is unable to begin until you have a current patient list and your consultant is frustrated as he needs to begin an all-day endoscopy list.

Rank in order the following actions in response to this situation (1 = Most appropriate; 5 = Least appropriate)

A Express your frustration with the IT equipment and demand that the consultant requests replacements.

B Send the patient list to your personal email address and print it on the neighbouring ward.

C Ask a medical student to print the list while you begin the ward round.

D Ask the nurses on each of the wards whether there are any new patients who are under the care of your consultant.

E Advise the team to reconvene in 15 minutes while you contact the IT helpdesk and attempt to print the list.

29. You observe an FY1 colleague shouting at a staff nurse in front of a patient. Afterwards, the nurse approaches you to discuss the FY1's behaviour. He explains that the FY1 has had several 'angry outbursts' since joining the ward two months ago, and he is unsure how to deal with them.

Rank in order the following actions in response to this situation (1 = Most appropriate; 5 = Least appropriate)

A Advise the nurse to talk to his line manager as it is not your responsibility to get involved in nursing-related matters.

B Bleep the FY1 and ask him to return to the ward and apologize to the nurse and patient.

C Apologize on behalf of the FY1, and ask the nurse not to pursue the matter any further at this time as you will speak to the other doctor.

D Inform the FY1 colleague's Clinical Supervisor about the episode and what the staff nurse has told you.

E Send an email to your FY1 colleague detailing what the staff nurse has told you, to provide a written record of your conversation.

30. During the return flight from your holiday abroad, an announcement is made requesting medical assistance for one of the passengers. You graduated from medical school three weeks ago and have yet to start your first job as an FY1 doctor; you feel particularly apprehensive about attending to a possible in-flight emergency on your own.

Rank in order the following actions in response to this situation (1 = Most appropriate; 5 = Least appropriate)

A Do nothing since you are not legally bound to provide medical assistance as you have not yet signed a contract with your employer.

B Inform the cabin crew that you are a recently qualified doctor, and begin your medical assessment immediately.

C Approach the unwell passenger and determine if you will be able to offer any help before informing the cabin crew of your presence.

D Wait for 10 minutes to see if anyone else on board can assist before volunteering to assess the passenger.

E Review the passenger, but ask the cabin crew to make an announcement for more senior medical assistance as you are only recently qualified and very inexperienced.

31. A group of medical students ask if you can help them prepare for their forthcoming end-of-module examination on the respiratory system. You agree to teach them at the end of the week, provided that they stay and assist you with some ward jobs that evening, which they agree to do. You are reminded about your teaching commitment the day before the students' examination, but unfortunately you have forgotten to prepare a relevant lesson plan.

Rank in order the following actions in response to this situation (1 = Most appropriate; 5 = Least appropriate)

A Inform the students that they should have reminded you earlier in the week, and now you are unable to teach them.

B Defer the teaching until they want to prepare for their next end-of-module examination.

C Attempt to teach the students, even if your knowledge is insufficient, but finish the teaching early if it does not prove helpful.

D Teach the students about haemotology, with which you are more comfortable.

E Adopt a style of teaching which only utilizes questioning the students, and reflect every question asked back towards the group.

32. You are asked by your consultant in paediatric surgery to clerk an infant who has been admitted to A&E with bilious vomiting. This is the first week of your first FY1 rotation and you have had limited experience in paediatrics beyond your five-week rotation in medical school two years ago. You are unsure whether you should clerk the patient, if you should inform the parents of your inexperience, and who would be responsible if you were to assess the infant.

Choose the THREE most appropriate actions to take in this situation

A Attempt a rudimentary clerking before calling the consultant to review the patient.

B Refuse to clerk the patient, on the grounds that you do not have sufficient experience.

C Conduct a thorough assessment of the patient once you are sure that he is stable.

D Act with the knowledge that the consultant is ultimately responsible for your assessment, as his trainee.

E Act with the knowledge that you are responsible for your assessment of the patient.

F Introduce yourself as a doctor, but do not state your seniority for fear of further worrying the infant's parents.

G State your position as a junior doctor.

H Admit that this is your first week as a junior doctor but that you will not be responsible for any treatment decisions yourself.

33. The final-year medical student attached to your ward asks you if you could write a reference in support of his application for a university-level history course which starts three months before his final-year examinations. You are concerned as, despite his enthusiasm, the student has a poor clinical knowledge base. You are not convinced by his assurances that he will be able to balance this new commitment with his medical course.

Rank in order the following actions in response to this situation
(1 = Most appropriate; 5 = Least appropriate)

A Write a reference indicating that his knowledge base is poor but that he might do much better in another academic subject.

B Write a supportive reference, as his clinical knowledge base is not relevant to his performance on a history course.

C Suggest that he asks your consultant to write a reference to provide a more seasoned perspective on his ability.

D Tell the student that your position might not qualify you to comment on his suitability for the course.

E Set the student a mock clinical examination, and offer to write his reference based on his performance.

34. A male FY1 colleague in paediatrics is clerking a frightened 15-year-old girl who has been brought into A&E by her older sister who says that she has been the victim of a violent attack. After establishing a good rapport with the patient, the FY1 arranges for a physical examination. However, the girl remains adamant that no one else be present. In the absence of your registrar, your fellow FY1 asks for your advice.

Rank in order the following actions in response to this situation
(1 = Most appropriate; 5 = Least appropriate)

A Advise him not to examine the patient and instead wait for the registrar.

B Suggest that he performs a physical examination by inspection alone, with a chaperone present if the girl agrees.

C He should agree to forego the chaperone and complete a thorough physical and internal examination to rule out any genital injury.

D Tell him to insist on the presence of a female nurse as a chaperone, and to avoid examining the patient if she insists on no one else being present.

E Ask the older sister to sign in the medical notes agreeing to act as the chaperone.

35. Your hospital is at the centre of a news story regarding a leaked audit which shows a recent rise in mortality following heart valve replacements. As an FY1 on the cardiothoracic ward, you feel strongly about the negative portrayal of your senior surgical colleagues' abilities, believing the results to be due to the use of a new prosthesis. A news reporter approaches you as you are leaving the ward and asks if you would like to comment.

Rank in order the following actions in response to this situation (1 = Most appropriate; 5 = Least appropriate)

A Share with the reporter your honest opinions of the competence of your senior colleagues and the possibility of a fault with the new prosthetic valves.

B Ask for the contact details of the reporter and agree to an interview once you have obtained permission from your local Trust.

C Politely decline to comment.

D Discuss in general terms the difficulty that surgical innovators face when introducing novel technologies, without going into specific details about your department.

E Explain your frustration with the ignorance demonstrated by the media and the general public in relation to health matters.

36. You have volunteered to be the deanery's FY1 representative. A recent survey has shown that the greatest frustration of 90% of FY1 doctors is the limited teaching given during a typical week. However, a senior member of the deanery committee has described his frustration at your 'difficult predecessor' who was constantly 'trying to change things', and you are unsure how receptive the committee will be to your suggestions.

Rank in order the following actions in response to this situation (1 = Most appropriate; 5 = Least appropriate)

A Based on the recent survey findings, request approval for a full review into the teaching provided for FY1 doctors by each hospital's postgraduate medical education office.

B Conduct another questionnaire asking more specific questions about the teaching to the FY1 doctors themselves.

C Avoid the topic during your initial committee meetings, as you are unlikely to gain the favour of your superiors.

D Predict the response of all of the FY1 doctors to questions on the failures of teaching based on your own experiences, and take this evidence to the committee as justification for a detailed review by each hospital's education office.

E Resign as the deanery's FY1 representative.

37. You receive a gift of substantial value from the family of a wealthy patient whom you have recently cared for on the ward. You are frequently praised for the time and effort which you spend with patients, but this is the first time that you have personally received a gift.

Rank in order the following actions in response to this situation (1 = Most appropriate; 5 = Least appropriate)

A Inform the GMC of the gift.

B Inform the Ward Sister in charge of the gift.

C Seek the advice of your medico-legal defence organization.

D Accept the gift, but share its monetary value with the rest of your medical team.

E Attempt to obtain the family's details and return the gift.

38. An FY1 who works with you on the surgical ward is asked to complete a death certificate and cremation form for a patient he has been treating. However, he has a conscientious objection to cremation, based on religious beliefs, and would prefer you to complete the form even though you have never met the patient.

Rank in order the following actions in response to this situation (1 = Most appropriate; 5 = Least appropriate)

A Agree to complete the cremation form, as your colleague has provided a valid reason for refusing.

B Advise your colleague to claim that he has not been adequately trained to complete cremation forms.

C Inform your colleague that he has a duty to put aside any personal beliefs and complete the cremation form.

D Suggest that the FY1 speaks to the bereaved family members and reminds them of the option of burial.

E Refuse to sign the cremation forms on the grounds that you are not familiar with the patient.

39. You are a foundation doctor with an interest in orthopaedic surgery. In an effort to improve your specialty training application, you would like to complete an Advanced Trauma Life Support (ATLS) course. Unfortunately, your Trust gives priority to doctors working in A&E. One of the A&E doctors has been given a place on this basis but offers it to you in exchange for covering one of his night shifts.

Rank in order the following actions in response to this situation
(1 = Most appropriate; 5 = Least appropriate)

A Accept the offer as it appears to be a mutually beneficial agreement.

B Tell the other foundation doctor that you will gratefully accept his offer but you are not willing to complete the weekend shift.

C Refuse the offer.

D Ask the advice of the ATLS coordinator at your hospital.

E Accept his offer and attend the course, but do not turn up for the weekend shift.

40. As the FY1 in cardiology, you are responsible for looking after your consultant's NHS patients. One of the patients who had been under your care for the last 48 hours is transferred to the private ward on the other side of the hospital. At the request of your consultant, the nurses on the private ward have bleeped you on several occasions to complete various clinical procedures. You feel challenged by the additional workload and are uncertain whether you will complete your routine tasks.

Rank in order the following actions in response to this situation
(1 = Most appropriate; 5 = Least appropriate)

A Ask the consultant for additional reimbursement in return for providing more of your time for assisting with his private patients.

B Explain the situation to one of the other cardiology consultants.

C Speak to the patient and ask whether he would mind returning to the NHS ward.

D Arrange a meeting with the cardiology consultant, via his secretary, to discuss the additional workload.

E Do not respond to any bleeps from the private ward; if it is genuinely a consultant's request he will contact you.

ANSWERS

1. **C, B, D, A, E**

Confidentiality is important for maintaining patient dignity and trust in the medical profession. The security of a patient list cannot be guaranteed at home and most Trusts will have policies preventing staff from removing details in this form. In the first instance, you should raise this informally with your colleague (C) and make policy easier to follow by asking for an appropriate waste container (B). If your colleague persists, you should escalate the problem appropriately (D). You should not discourage your colleague from knowing the patients better if your motive is competition (A). This would not foster a culture of excellence and may lead to conflict. You should not be tempted to behave inappropriately because others are doing so (E).

2. **B, E, D, C, A**

Although all patient information is confidential, particularly sensitive details may warrant a higher level of security. You should avoid including such details routinely (e.g. on patient lists) if possible (B). Otherwise, you should respect the principles of confidentiality as for all your patients (E). Although errors are possible, you should be sufficiently certain of maintaining confidentiality that you can strongly reassure the patient (D). Invasive procedures should be performed safely regardless of whether the patient is known to have a blood-borne illness. Colleagues do not routinely need to know about HIV status (C) as this should not change their practice. However, an HIV diagnosis is an important context with implications for diagnosis and management of other conditions. Therefore this detail must appear in the permanent patient record (A).

3. **A, C, D, E, B**

This group is exposing patient confidentiality to significant risk. You should first let the group know that they can be overheard by speaking to individuals (A) or to the group as a whole (C). If the breach is significant or cannot be abated, you should raise the issue formally with the Trust (D). Although staff are responsible for their own actions, you have a professional duty to protect patients and challenge inappropriate behaviour (E). Hospital security is unlikely to have a role away from the hospital site (B).

4. **A, B, C, E, D**

You have a duty to take appropriate action following any concerns about patient care, dignity, or safety. If patient dignity is currently under threat, appropriate action might require intervening at that time (A). The GMC requires that concerns are raised with an 'appropriate officer' of the organization, which will depend on their specific nature. This person might be in the nursing hierarchy (B) or a senior manager (e.g. clinical governance lead). You should not make preliminary enquiries unless absolutely necessary as this might obstruct a formal investigation (C).

Concerns should not be raised externally unless you have exhausted internal procedures without success (E). The GMC imposes a *duty* on doctors to raise concerns about patient dignity being compromised. You are not at liberty to ignore this event (D).

5. C, E, D, B, A

The GMC is clear that doctors must not sign contracts which fetter their ability to raise concerns. You should explain this politely but firmly (C). If in doubt, the GMC or a medical defence organization might be able to help (E). You should avoid signing any guarantee in the knowledge that you will breach it if necessary (D). However, the law will void agreements intended to stop employees making disclosures about health or safety. Simply disposing of the agreement (B) ignores the inappropriate requirement and may lead to employment difficulties later on. You should certainly not sign an agreement of this nature intending to be bound (A) as this is contrary to your professional obligations.

6. C, A, B, D, E

Although the diagnosis might be clear, you are responsible for the appropriateness of prescriptions and should review the patient yourself (C), (A). Antibiotic policies will reflect local resistance patterns and should be followed unless there are good clinical reasons to depart from protocol (B).

There is no good reason why a nurse should not test urine (D) subject to the same restrictions as any other health professional(e.g. patient consent). It is important to treat patients before they become haemodynamically compromised and not afterwards (E).

7. A, B, E, D, C

It is not sufficient to simply raise concerns; you must be satisfied that they have been appropriately acted upon. If concerns are not resolved, these must be escalated as far up the Trust hierarchy as necessary (A). You should document each stage carefully (B). Although you must 'do your best' under the circumstances, you should avoid ignoring structural problems (E). You should not generally take concerns externally, unless through appropriate channels (e.g. the GMC, the Care Quality Commission) after internal processes have been exhausted. Raising issues related to a specific hospital in the press may leave you open to disciplinary action by your employer (D). In addition, a hidden camera (C) would betray the confidence of patients and colleagues and seriously harm trust in the medical profession.

8. B, C, A, D, E

External courses can be useful for professional development and should be attended if possible (C).

The most appropriate option would be to gather support from your Clinical or Educational Supervisor and then approach the manager with responsibility for workforce planning in your department (B). If you are entitled to time off in lieu (because of working late on other days), a special arrangement may be possible. However, you should not unilaterally decide that you are entitled to attend the course (D).

It may be tempting to arrange informal cover with other members of your team (A). However, this may breach departmental rules and problems could arise, for example if that team member is deployed elsewhere because of staff shortages or is unwell on the day in question.

Although consultants lead the clinical team, it is often insufficient to have their agreement alone (E). Your consultant's support may be very influential in determining the final decision, but other people (e.g. the Medical Staffing manager) should be involved in a decision of this kind.

9. C, B, D, A, E

You should discuss any issues raised to clarify misunderstandings (C) and put right anything you are able to. It may be helpful to direct the patient to PALS who can offer advice independently of the clinical team (B). You should inform the medical and nursing hierarchy of any concerns so that these can be rectified and a complaint anticipated (D). Although you should certainly resolve concerns if possible, you must not discourage others (including relatives) from raising concerns about patient care (A). However, you should not aggravate the situation, particularly by indicating that specific colleagues are to blame (E).

10. A, D, C, B, E

Your first priority is Tim's safety. Therefore you must ensure that he does not receive the drug by stopping the prescription and informing the nurse (A). A note should be clear on the drug chart and notes so that similar prescription errors are avoided in future (D). The prescriber should be told so that they can amend their practice and also in case they had a good reason for their action (C). Although no harm came to the patient, this is a 'near miss' and a clinical incident form should be completed (B). Stopping the prescription is your priority, but other actions must be taken to reduce the risk of this happening again (E).

11. C, E, H

The GMC imposes a duty to raise concerns about patient safety. However, if you are uncertain how to proceed, the GMC suggests getting advice from a senior member of staff (H), a GMC employer liaison adviser (E), a medical defence organization (C), or Public Concern at Work, which is a charity providing confidential advice in such cases. The absent consultant (A), moonlighting SHO (G), and the consultant opposed to private practice seem (F) unlikely sources of impartial advice. Your partner (B) and friend from school (D) are not recommended as they might not understand the issues and/or might not be bound by professional duty (e.g. to keep your concerns in confidence).

12. B, D, H

All doctors should encourage a culture in which concerns can be raised openly. This is particularly important for medical students who must learn early on not to ignore concerns. However, you should seek to clarify any misunderstandings and mention that consent might have been obtained without the student being present (B). Ultimately, the student should raise this issue with the consultant (D) to ensure they are not complicit in examining patients inappropriately. If they have concerns, their medical school will have its own 'raising concerns' policy (H). You should not advise the student to keep quiet about their concerns (A) (C) (E). Specific consent for examination by medical students cannot be implied by consent to an operation (F). Raising the concern anonymously (G) may be unhelpful, as misunderstandings cannot be clarified and neither can further details be gathered for the concern to be acted upon. The student may wish to contact his medical school (H) before escalating concerns up the Trust hierarchy.

13. B, E, D

As a doctor, you have a responsibility to maintain your clinical skills and learn from patients. It is important to make allowance for this despite routine clinical commitments (F). Educational opportunities should be recognized for their intrinsic value and not simply to gain work-based assessments (H). This case clearly raises an issue of consent which is impossible to obtain under the circumstances. However, you are unlikely to feel a ruptured abdominal aortic aneurysm in a well patient and a brief abdominal examination may be appropriate (D) (A). As a doctor, you are in a different position from medical students who cannot directly influence a patient's care (C). If you were to examine the patient, it might be appropriate to ask the senior clinician responsible for their care (E). However, calling the patient's relatives at a time when they are probably distraught is likely to be unhelpful (G). You should certainly identify this gap in your experience and read about aneurysms whether or not you examine the patient (B).

14. A, E, F

Work-based assessments are only one means of developing your clinical skills as a doctor. You may wish to examine every patient formally as if you were being observed and assessed (F). You might also gain by presenting and/or discussing the case (A). In this instance, the 'helpful' SHO might agree to watch you examine the patient before completing the assessment (E). Delaying the patient's assessment or care for your benefit is unacceptable (G).

Nevertheless, it is important to recognize that senior doctors have other commitments and cannot always be available to teach. Reminding the medical registrar of their teaching responsibilities is unlikely to nurture a joyous teacher–student relationship (B). Although assessments can be difficult to obtain, each trainee is responsible for achieving a minimum number (H).

You should resist offers from other doctors to complete work-based assessments if the criteria for these have not been satisfied (C) (D). These offers jeopardize the probity of senior doctors and may deprive you of opportunities for genuine feedback.

15. **A, D, E**

It is your responsibility to satisfy all mandatory requirements of the Foundation Programme. However, foundation doctors are a key part of the clinical team and your absence could impact negatively on patient care. Therefore you should take steps to minimize the impact of your absence.

You should attend mandatory commitments (A) unless this compromises patient safety. However, to resolve a potential conflict in future, you should seek advice from your consultant (D). It should be possible for another member of your team (e.g. the SHO or registrar) to lead the ward round (E) in your absence and you can update this person to facilitate continuity of patient care. Only extraordinary circumstances should cause you to miss teaching (C) (F). If you have to miss a mandatory training session (e.g. because of a clinical emergency) you should ensure that you catch up in other ways, such as private study (G).

Signing the attendance register dishonestly (B) or asking someone else to do so (H) raises significant probity issues.

16. **E, F, H**

Doctors have a duty to promote the education and development of junior colleagues. You should accept your consultant's request unless patient care is likely to suffer by doing so (A). You should be frank with your consultant so that he can make alternative arrangements if you cannot help (C). Signing students' attendance forms before sending them away (B) deprives them of teaching and casts doubt on your own probity.

A formal tutorial might be useful, but under these circumstances might conflict with ward commitments (D). You should seek context from the students (E) and assign clear tasks which help your workload (e.g. cannulation) if possible (F). However, you should not ask them to spend significant amounts of time on routine tasks with limited educational value (G). When teaching students, try to strike a balance between topics which are useful and those with which you are familiar (H).

17. **A, E, F**

You must be open and honest while delivering feedback in a constructive and professional manner. Raising your concerns throughout the placement (A) (B) will allow the student to explain his behaviour (F) and adjust his attitude.

It would be dishonest to mark the student as 'satisfactory' in a domain if you actually believe otherwise (C). Instead, you should raise your concerns using specific examples (E) as when giving any negative feedback. However, concerns should only be raised with the Clinical Supervisor (D) or medical school (G) if their gravity warrants such interventions. Inciting the nursing staff to prejudge the incoming FY1 (H) would be unhelpful and make it harder for him to change before starting the post.

18. C, D, F

Doctors must continue to develop knowledge throughout their careers and ensure that they are up to date. You should either ask for time during the day to complete the modules (C) or recognize their general benefit and do so at home (D). Refusing to comply with reasonable requests from your Trust (A) (E) (H) may cause employment difficulties.

Asking someone else to complete the modules (G) or doing so without reading their content (B) deprives them of their educational purpose. The former is also dishonest.

Whether or not you found the modules helpful, you should consider providing feedback (F) so that they can be developed and improved for others.

19. C, D, G

You should avoid compromising your professional relationship with colleagues, including medical students (H). As a doctor on the team, you are responsible for their supervision, learning, and continued assessment. Attention should not be distributed unfairly (C) and romantic relationships should be discouraged (D), ideally at the earliest possible stage (G).

It would be unhelpful and unfair to avoid one particular student (A) and unprofessional to meet socially with ulterior motives (B). Although honesty is usually commendable, a frank discussion should be avoided (E) as it risks escalating the situation and surprising the student, particularly if you have misinterpreted their feelings. Similarly, asking questions of other students should be avoided (F).

20. B, F, H

There is no absolute rule preventing doctors from accepting gifts. However, the GMC does prohibit doctors from inviting or pressuring patients to make gifts, either to themselves or to anyone else. For this reason, you should not suggest that Sid donates money to a specific charity (G) or that he offers you a different amount (A).

Many Trusts will have policies on gifts (e.g. a maximum value) with which you should be familiar before accepting (H), and not afterwards (C). Although rules will vary, explaining that you are unable to accept the gift (B) is certainly an acceptable response. At the very least, you should not accept a high-value gift immediately without being convinced that it is more than a spontaneous gesture (F).

Transferring money from the patient to his daughter (E) when this was not its intention would be inappropriate. Asking Sid to sign a statement (D) would overly formalize the situation and not protect you against the accusation of having coerced the gift. If you feel that this is necessary given the gift's high value, this is an indicator that the gift is inappropriate.

21. C, D, F

In this dilemma, you must balance the principles of autonomy and non-maleficence. *Good Medical Practice* reminds us that 'doctors must not discriminate against patients by allowing personal views to adversely affect the professional relationship with patients or the treatment they provide' (A). The patient has severe post-partum haemorrhage (PPH) and a transfusion is indicated, but it cannot be given without consent. There is no risk to the life of the child (B). It is essential to confirm the patient's wishes and clarify with certainty any decision to refuse blood products (C) before ruling out a transfusion (D), and it should not be assumed that her wishes would be consistent with 'typical' Jehovah's Witness practice. It would be unethical to transfuse the patient without frank discussion while she remains conscious (E). In complex cases involving Jehovah's Witnesses it is absolutely essential to involve senior colleagues, and a haematologist should also be involved early on (F). If the patient agrees to their involvement, a Jehovah's Witness Hospital Liaison Committee can serve as a useful source of support for patients (G). There is no suggestion that the patient currently lacks the capacity to make a decision (H).

22. B, A, D, E, C

As the admitting doctor you may be the only qualified professional to perform a detailed physical examination, and you should ensure that you clearly document all your findings (B). Although it might not be directly relevant to the current presentation (A), it would be sensible to discuss any concerns you have with your seniors. At some stage it may be necessary to surgically correct the circumcision; however, any assessment and subsequent referral should be made by a senior (D). The assessment of a child's best interests must include the cultural/religious values of the child and/or parents (E), and members of certain religious communities consider male circumcision fundamental to their religious practice (C). However, female genital circumcision (or mutilation) is usually a criminal offence and a serious child protection issue.

23. E, D, C, B, A

GMC guidance reminds us that probity is at the heart of medical professionalism. In this instance, it is important to address the issues of erroneous payment for locum shifts and working additional unpaid hours separately. The immediate priority should be to return any excess payment to your employer (E) before seeking to rectify your own excessive working hours, which may benefit from the input of your Educational Supervisor (D). At some stage it may become necessary to formally document your additional work hours in a work diary (C). It would certainly be a moral hazard to retain any percentage of money, however small, belonging to your employer (B). Even if it became evident that you had worked a similar number of hours unpaid, failure to raise the issue would cast serious doubt on your professional judgment (A). It could also lead to disciplinary or even legal action.

24. B, D, F

This scenario tests honesty about experiences and qualifications when applying for posts. The GMC requires that relevant information must not be deliberately omitted. While it is possible mislead the reader with sentences which imply particular experiences (e.g. theatre exposure (A) (E) and courses attended (G)), it would be more honest to describe actual experiences on the ward (B) and alternative means of learning about operations (D), and to share your enthusiasm for future training (F). Arguments about too few opportunities (C) or unjustified claims of superior clinical competence (H) are unlikely to impress a selection panel.

25. E, C, B, D, A

Integrity is an essential foundation for any clinical or scientific study, including audit, which rests on the honesty and openness of the investigators. Conclusions must not be reached hastily from findings which may be misinterpreted. Preoperative parameters (e.g. older patients) might explain the differences and should be explored (E). If this fails to explain the differences, the consultant should be offered an opportunity to consider the findings (C). It would be discourteous and unprofessional to approach his colleagues first in such an open forum (B). You must not manipulate data to give a misleading impression for any reason (D). Reporting the surgeon to an external body should never be a first step or one taken lightly (A), as this risks serious anxiety and unqualified reputational damage to the consultant, and to yourself if the allegations were found to be unfair.

26. D, F, H

The GMC sets out professional standards which guide undergraduate medical students (A). Behaviour outside the clinical environment can impact on a student's fitness to practise and should always justify public trust in the medical profession. The students should be asked to explain their actions (A). It is unlikely to be resolved at the time of the incident (B) and is not the responsibility of your own supervisors (C). Instead, the students should be confronted soon after the incident (F) (G) and their supervisors informed of this breach of professional duty (D). Informing your colleagues is unlikely to improve the situation (H). The police will deal with the students in their own way—your responsibilities as a member of the medical profession are different (E).

27. D, C, E, B, A

According to *Good Medical Practice*, doctors must inform the GMC without delay if they have 'accepted a caution, been charged or found guilty of a criminal offence, anywhere in the world' (D). This includes motoring offences unless these are resolved by a fixed penalty notice. Medical defence organizations can provide legal advice and support in fitness to practise cases, and it might be prudent to inform your medical defence organization (C). Your consultant should provide advice already available to you in Good Medical Practice (E). It would be contrary to guidelines to delay informing the GMC either temporarily (B) or indefinitely (A).

28. E, C, D, A, B

Punctuality is an essential attribute for facilitating expeditious patient care. In this instance, a delay in printing the patient list has limited the team available to review each patient. Resolving the matter yourself appears to be the fastest and fairest approach (E). A medical student should not usually be handed responsibility for something you are struggling to achieve yourself (C). Alternative means of identifying your patients could result in prolonging the ward round and risks missing individuals under your care (D). It would be unproductive and inappropriate to make demands on your consultant at this time (A). It is never appropriate to use personal email addresses to send patient information (B).

29. D, B, A, E, C

Doctors must treat colleagues fairly and with respect. GMC guidance on respecting colleagues prohibits bullying and unfounded criticism that might undermine patients' trust in their care. The nature of this episode, and the frequency with which it has reportedly occurred, requires senior involvement, e.g. your colleague's Clinical Supervisor (D). Approaching the FY1 immediately after the outburst (B) may antagonize your colleague and is unlikely to result in a satisfactory outcome. Emailing the FY1 with the nurse's comments (E) does create a written record but could be open to misinterpretation. The situation could benefit from your apology but you should not attempt to silence your nursing colleague (C). Although the nurse may well choose to consult a senior, you should not derogate all responsibility if approached by a colleague with concerns (A).

30. B, E, C, D, A

The GMC requires that 'in an emergency, wherever it arises, you must offer assistance, taking account of your own safety, competence, and the availability of other options for care'. (B) As a recently qualified doctor, it would be difficult to justify ignoring the call for help, irrespective of a legal requirement to act (A) Declaring your inexperience may encourage others to attend, but could wait until your assessment suggests that further help is required (E). Although you should work within your limits, inexperience is a poor reason for failing to act appropriately in an emergency (C) (D).

31. C, E, D, B, A

Doctors must be willing to teach and train students and other doctors as part of their responsibility for the care of patients now and in the future. This requirement requires the appropriate skills and attitudes of an effective teacher, one of which is effective planning. In failing to prepare, you risk providing ineffective teaching and failing to impart relevant knowledge or skills (E), or to meet the learning objectives of your students (D). It would be unjust not to attempt any teaching which the students might find useful (B, A). The best response in this scenario is to begin your unprepared teaching with a willingness to conclude early if it is not proving useful (C).

32. **C, E, G**

As a foundation doctor, you will experience many practices for the first time (B), and the safe management of patients should be paramount (A). You should use an ABCDE approach and ensure that all patients are stable before completing a more thorough assessment (C). You are ultimately responsible for your actions when assessing and treating any patient (E), while the consultant takes responsibility for your training and supervision (D). In introducing yourself to a patient or parents, you are clarifying your position within the team of doctors providing their care (G) (F). Your introduction does not require a detailed account of your training and experiences as this may unduly compromise the trust placed in your advice (H). However, it is important to remain honest and transparent if asked about your grade or experience by the patient's family.

33. **D, C, E, A, B**

References should be written honestly and objectively, particularly with respect to positions in healthcare which may place patients at risk if individuals are appointed incorrectly. As a junior doctor providing informal supervision, you may not be best placed to provide a reference (D). Your consultant may be able to provide a more experienced and meaningful perspective (C). The major concern in this case is the impact a new commitment would have on this student's final examinations. If your doubts about the student's abilities are ambiguous, you could set an objective test on which a reference might be based (E). However, as a relatively junior doctor, you should be cautious before providing a definitive statement as to whether or not the student is likely to balance the two commitments (A) (B).

34. **D, B, E, A, C**

Although the FY1 has commendably established rapport with the patient, he is still obliged to offer a chaperone during the physical examination. In some circumstances, a male doctor should insist on a chaperone being present for his own protection (C) (D). A young person who is potentially vulnerable after a serious physical or sexual assault would be one such case. If the patient disagrees, a limited examination with a chaperone in attendance might be justifiable (B). The older sister could act as a chaperone but a female colleague would be preferable (E). Although the FY1 should ensure that there are no life-threatening injuries, an internal examination in this case requires additional experience and should be repeated as few times as possible. Thus it may be left to a more senior doctor (A).

35. **C, B, D, A, E**

Even as a more junior doctor, it is essential to realize the impact that your comments can have on your own hospital and more widely across the profession itself, particularly those made available in the public domain. In a scenario such as this, where the issue is likely to be the subject of an active investigation, it might be prudent to avoid (C) or at least delay (B) any personal comments, particularly those which could be misconstrued as representing the hospital or doctors in question. While it may be possible to share your general thoughts about related issues (D), there remains a risk of false inferences being made as to the position of the hospital. In sharing your personal opinion you risk incriminating a manufacturer's product based on only limited information, which could have significant legal consequences for yourself and your Trust (A). Finally, using this opportunity to lambast the public's knowledge on health issues is unlikely to promote confidence and trust in the medical profession (E).

36. **B, A, C, E, D**

In accepting this position you have made a commitment to represent your foundation colleagues and convey their concerns to the deanery's committee. However, it is also necessary to make the appropriate request to the committee, and in this instance more information about the FY1 doctor's concerns should probably be established first (B). Requesting a full review at this time based on one survey statistic provides less convincing justification for your request (A) and may worsen the situation between yourself and the senior committee member, although it is an attempt at resolving the problem of the poor teaching. It is certainly not acceptable to ignore the issue in an effort to gain favour (C), but at least it may mean that the problem can be addressed at a later date. Therefore C is better than D or E. You might decide to resign; however, having accepted the position, making a difficult request should not be beyond the foundation doctor (E) and this does not produce any solution to the problem at all. It would never be acceptable to present falsified data, regardless of your intention (D), and this raises issues of probity.

37. **E, C, B, A, D**

You must never encourage patients or their relatives to offer gifts that will directly or indirectly benefit you, and you should make reasonable efforts to dissuade them from such offers (E). It is sensible to seek advice from a medico-legal organization when accepting a gift of high value (C). The most immediate source of advice might be the Ward Sister (B), but your service manager or consultant might also know about local policy with respect to gifts. Informing the GMC might be necessary if you were unable to return a high-value gift (A). Retaining the gift without seeking advice or declaring its existence is the least favourable option (D).

38. **E, C, B, D, A**

All qualified doctors have a legal obligation to sign cremation forms, and cannot refuse on personal or religious objections to cremation (Cremation Acts 1902 and 1952). In instances where you are the only doctor able to legally sign the form, refusal to do so could cause unnecessary delay and distress to the relatives. In this case, you should state up front that you are unable to complete the form, having never met the patient (E), and suggest that your colleague put aside his objections (C).

Clearly, it is inappropriate to suggest that your colleague lies about his abilities (B) or interferes with the wishes of a bereaved family (D). You cannot complete the cremation form as you do not satisfy the requirement of knowing the patient (A).

39. **D, C, B, A, E**

Although you are keen to attend the course, it would be wrong to subvert the process for allocating places. If your colleague is unable to attend the course, he should explain this to the coordinators. Therefore you should ask whether they would agree to transfer the place to you from your colleague (D). Alternatively, you should decline the offer as the place could be re-allocated more equitably (C).

The offer is further corrupted by the prospect of 'buying' and 'selling' a place which could have been used for a more appropriate candidate. It would be preferable to decline this part of the bargain if the 'spare' place was accepted (B) (A). Clearly, agreeing to cover a shift and then not turning up risks overburdening colleagues and compromising patient safety (E).

40. **D, B, C, A, E**

Your NHS employer has allocated a set amount of work per employee and may not have accounted for additional tasks on the private ward. Your primary responsibility is for your *own* patients and their care must not be compromised by acquiescence to inappropriate requests, even if driven by your consultant. You should talk to the consultant first (D) before seeking the advice of other senior colleagues (B). It would be inappropriate to speak directly to the patient, particularly about moving their care back to the NHS (C).

Seeking additional pay for time already compensated by your NHS employer would be dishonest (A). You should always answer your bleep if contacted, as the next request might be reasonable or impact on patient safety (E).

Coping with pressure

Introduction

Questions within this section will explore your resilience and ability to work under pressure. Through your responses, you will need to demonstrate a willingness to remain flexible, manage ambiguity, and adapt to changing circumstances.

The ability to remain calm while handling stressful situations arising with patients, relatives, and colleagues is of the utmost importance. Problems must be resolved directly but may require a diplomatic approach to avoid conflict. It is therefore important to speak to others respectfully, seek help early on, and remain aware of your own limitations.

- However many demands are made on your time, you must prioritize to ensure that the most important tasks are completed first.
- Patients who are haemodynamically unstable are your first priority. Those in pain or distress are second. Routine tasks (e.g. discharge summaries) can wait until an appropriate moment.
- If you are not coping with your workload to the detriment of patients, you must summon assistance. If help is not available, it should be escalated to a senior.

QUESTIONS

1. You are a new FY1 on an orthopaedic team. The morning ward round is running late and both your consultant and registrar need to go to theatre. One patient has yet to be consented for a hemiarthroplasty after fracturing her hip. Your registrar tells you to make sure that she is consented in time to be second on the morning list.

Rank in order the following actions in response to this situation
(1 = Most appropriate; 5 = Least appropriate)

A Consent the patient before doing any other jobs.

B Complete all urgent jobs arising from the ward round, and then consent the patient.

C Explain that you are not sufficiently experienced to consent patients for this operation.

D Ask an SHO from another team who can perform hip hemiarthroplasties to take consent.

E Agree to consent the patient and then ask experienced nurses to show you how to do this correctly.

2. You are the FY1 on call for medicine. After seeing a patient with pancreatitis, you recall the need to take an arterial blood gas (ABG). Unfortunately your only experience of this procedure was on a model two years previously. You have never attempted to perform an ABG on a patient before and are not feeling confident about success.

Rank in order the following actions in response to this situation
(1 = Most appropriate; 5 = Least appropriate)

A Call the duty medical registrar and ask them to supervise your first ABG.

B Ask another FY1 who is more confident with procedures to help.

C Attempt the procedure but without warning the patient about your inexperience.

D Wait until the end of your shift and then hand the job over to the night team.

E Attempt the procedure twice after talking to the patient, and then ask for help if unsuccessful.

3. As the FY1 on call you are bleeped by the pathology laboratory about an abnormal blood result. They give you a value representing severe hypernatraemia. You do not recall very much about hypernatraemia and have never managed a patient with this problem before.

Rank in order the following actions in response to this situation
(1 = Most appropriate; 5 = Least appropriate)

A Call the duty medical registrar and ask what to do.

B See the patient to check that they are well, and then call the duty medical registrar.

C Find a computer terminal and Google 'hypernatraemia' for inspiration.

D Consult hospital guidelines, either in paper form or online.

E Prescribe a loop diuretic such as furosemide.

4. You are on a busy surgical ward round. Your consultant tells you to order an urgent CT and make sure that it happens that morning. Although you make a note on your jobs list to do this, you do not think that there is a good reason for doing the scan.

Rank in order the following actions in response to this situation
(1 = Most appropriate; 5 = Least appropriate)

A Ask the consultant what the scan is for.

B Tell the duty radiologist that you disagree with doing the scan but have been told that it is urgent.

C Explain to your consultant you cannot order the scan as you disagree that it is appropriate.

D Ask a colleague in your team whether they can explain why the CT is necessary.

E Book an ultrasound instead and then reconsider the CT later depending on its results.

5. You are bleeped to Matron's office to discuss a prescribing error from your night shift the previous week. You prescribed a ten times overdose which fortunately was spotted by a vigilant pharmacist and never administered. Nevertheless, a clinical incident form has been completed and Matron is going to contact your Educational Supervisor. You feel that this error was caused by being overly tired.

Rank in order the following actions in response to this situation
(1 = Most appropriate; 5 = Least appropriate)

A Tell Matron that the error was not your fault because the Trust made you work unsafe hours.

B Accept personal responsibility but explain the factors which you believe contributed to the error.

C Ask Matron not to contact your Educational Supervisor as this was an isolated error.

D Use your e-portfolio to record the error and reflect on its reasons so as to avoid this happening again.

E Ask to meet your Educational Supervisor to discuss the error and your concerns about the night rota.

6. You are enjoying an evening meal with your friends when you remember ordering a blood test for an unwell patient, the result of which you forgot to check or hand over.

Rank in order the following actions in response to this situation
(1 = Most appropriate; 5 = Least appropriate)

A Make a note to check the result first thing in the morning before the ward round.

B Call the duty house officer through the switchboard and ask them to check the result.

C Put the issue out of your mind—it's important to 'turn off' after work.

D Reflect on how this test was missed and resolve to develop a system to ensure that such an error does not occur in the future.

E Drive back to the hospital to check the result yourself.

7. An FY1 doctor with whom you work closely says she is concerned that you seem 'down' and have been so for a few weeks. You have noticed that your mood is lower than normal but put this down to stress and tiredness. You do not think that you are clinically depressed and are embarrassed by your colleague raising the possibility.

Rank in order the following actions in response to this situation
(1 = Most appropriate; 5 = Least appropriate)

A Clarify the nature and reasons for your colleague's concern.

B See your Educational Supervisor at the next possible opportunity to discuss your mental health.

C Make a routine appointment with your GP.

D Ask other FY1 colleagues whether they think you are depressed.

E Use a depression screening tool to determine whether you are at risk.

8. After an emergency operation, a patient is left with a colostomy. You are the first doctor to see the patient once he becomes conversant, and he asks whether the bag is permanent. You are certain that colostomies can be reversed but do not remember very much else.

Rank in order the following actions in response to this situation
(1 = Most appropriate; 5 = Least appropriate)

A Tell the patient that his colostomy will be reversed.

B Explain that you are an FY1 and cannot answer complicated surgical questions.

C Explain that colostomies can sometimes be reversed and that you will help find out the plan in his case.

D Offer to ask your registrar to drop by later on to answer specific questions.

E Put time aside to read about stomas so you can answer questions more fully next time.

9. You are seeing a very unwell patient on your ward. He is complaining of chest pain and is also becoming increasingly hypotensive, despite fluid resuscitation. Over the previous few minutes, he has started to become drowsy. Although you are an FY1, you recently completed an Advanced Life Support (ALS) course and feel confident in managing acutely unwell patients.

Rank in order the following actions in response to this situation
(1 = Most appropriate; 5 = Least appropriate)

A Summon the resuscitation team.

B Use this case to consolidate ALS training, and then reflect on improving your management of acutely unwell patients.

C Give high-flow oxygen and more IV fluids.

D Call the SHO on her mobile phone for advice.

E Continue managing the patient unless he continues to deteriorate.

10. Your consultant asks you to meet her in her office. She tells you that she is concerned about your performance; specifically that you sometimes arrive late for her ward rounds and that your level of clinical knowledge is below her expectations of a doctor at your level. You disagree with this assessment, as you have only been late twice and do not think that there are any particular gaps in your knowledge.

Rank in order the following actions in response to this situation
(1 = Most appropriate; 5 = Least appropriate)

A Explain why you feel that her assessment is unfair, and ask her to provide specific examples to illustrate her concerns.

B Ask the foundation school about the possibility of changing consultants as there has been a relationship breakdown.

C Ask the consultant for advice about how you can act on her concerns and improve your performance.

D Using your e-portfolio, conduct a Team Assessment of Behaviour (TAB) round looking for evidence of concern about your performance from other colleagues.

E Tell the consultant that you believe your knowledge to be no worse than that of other FY1 doctors, and that you won several prizes at medical school.

11. You have always enjoyed alcohol and but recently have been drinking more than usual. There is no reason for you to think that this has affected your performance and you have never been drunk at work. However, a number of junior colleagues have commented on your alcohol intake, and one has told you that she is concerned that you are developing a dependency. As a result, you have begun to worry about your intake.

Choose the THREE most appropriate actions to take in this situation

A Ask a friend with whom you socialize whether he/she thinks that you are drinking too much.

B Ask other FY1 doctors not to joke about your drinking, as you feel that this undermines your professional reputation.

C Use a validated assessment tool (e.g. CAGE) to determine whether you have developed an alcohol problem.

D Make an appointment with your GP to discuss your concerns about your alcohol intake.

E Discuss the issue with your Educational Supervisor at your next meeting.

F Stop drinking for a week to see if you develop withdrawal symptoms.

G Think carefully about your reasons for drinking more than usual recently, and consider modifying your drinking pattern.

H Stop going out with colleagues and drink secretly instead to avoid damage to your reputation.

12. You have been working as an FY1 doctor for six weeks, but struggle with intravenous cannulation; in fact, you have yet to site one successfully despite several attempts. You are concerned about the distress caused to patients by your unsuccessful attempts and your inability to cannulate is starting to have an impact on the length of your working day.

Choose the THREE most appropriate actions to take in this situation

A Ask colleagues to site intravenous cannulas as often as possible until your ability improves.

B Using your e-portfolio, reflect on what it is that you are finding difficult about intravenous cannulation and how you can overcome this.

C Ask a senior colleague to supervise a series of cannulation attempts.

D Avoid trying to cannulate patients with 'difficult veins', and ask colleagues to see them instead.

E Consider modifying career aspirations to specialties which are less procedural.

F Continue to practise, recognizing that the procedure will become easier as you do.

G Attempt to cannulate each patient no more than once; if unsuccessful, bleep the duty anaesthetist for assistance.

H Tell every patient that they have 'difficult veins' so that their expectations of success are set low from the outset.

13. You are a lone FY1 seeing an elderly patient on the ward who is hypotensive despite being given intravenous fluids. You are con-cerned that the only intervention you know for managing hypotension has not worked in this case.

Choose the THREE most appropriate actions to take in this situation

A Ensure that the patient has a valid Not For Resuscitation order in case they suffer cardiac arrest.

B Accept that the patient is normally hypotensive and avoid further intravenous fluids.

C Call your SHO or other senior doctor for advice and assistance.

D Ask the nursing staff to put out a peri-arrest call.

E Begin administering inotropes if further fluid challenges fail to increase the blood pressure.

F Ask the patient's family to attend as their relative is probably dying.

G Ensure that you have good intravenous access and give another fluid challenge.

H Monitor the patient carefully for signs of deterioration.

14. You are feeling stressed as the on-call FY1 and have just found yourself becoming angry with two sets of relatives in quick succession.

Choose the THREE most appropriate actions to take in this situation

A Take a short break to regain perspective.

B Ask a colleague to help share your workload if they are able.

C Resolve not to speak with any more relatives on this shift as your priority must be unwell patients.

D Apologize to the relatives so that they are unlikely to complain.

E Consider what factors led to the altercations and address these as far as possible.

F Ask security or a nursing sister to remove the relatives so that you are not interrupted again.

G Manage your frustration by berating a medical student because he is unable to cannulate a patient.

H Check the time—it may nearly be time to go home.

15. Your manager emails to say that a written complaint has been received about your management of a patient seen in A&E. This concerns a patient whom you saw after a fall but did not document a proper examination. A fractured hip was missed for 72 hours.

Choose the THREE most appropriate actions to take in this situation

A Edit the notes to include features which you honestly recall at the time persuaded you that the patient did not have a broken hip.

B Edit the notes to include features which were not present but might make your mistake easier to forgive.

C Submit a factual description of events within the deadline imposed.

D Think honestly about the case and what you would do differently in future.

E Ignore the email as you are rotating to a new hospital next week.

F Explain that you were very busy that day and could not thoroughly examine every patient.

G Document your formal response and ask to be informed of the outcome of this complaint.

H Submit a response whenever you are able—the clinical care of your current patients comes first.

16. Your consultant calls to ask you to relocate a dislocated total hip replacement for a patient on the orthopaedic ward. He mentions that you should give intravenous sedation first. When you tell him that you have never sedated a patient before, he tells you to use propofol and ketamine, and then hangs up the phone.

Choose the THREE most appropriate actions to take in this situation

A Call the consultant back to clarify what doses you should use and what movements are necessary to replace the dislocated limb.

B Call the consultant back to say that you are unwilling to do as he asks.

C Use the *British National Formulary* to determine doses.

D Sedate the patient and then find the duty orthopaedic registrar if you are unable to relocate the dislocated hip.

E Contact your Educational Supervisor at the first possible opportunity to discuss this request.

F Contact another senior orthopaedic colleague if your consultant does not answer or offers no further advice.

G Attempt to relocate the hip without using sedation.

H Sedate the patient and attempt to relocate the hip.

17. A patient asks you why you are ordering a CT to eliminate stroke as a possible cause of her symptoms. She is worried about radiation risk and wants an MRI instead. You do not recall precisely why CT is used as the first-line investigation for stroke.

Choose the THREE most appropriate actions to take in this situation

A Tell her that CT is probably cheaper than MRI.

B Explain that you are a junior doctor and cannot answer questions about complex investigations.

C Call the duty radiologist and hand the phone to the patient so that they can have an informed discussion.

D Explain that you do not know the answer but will speak with someone to find out the reason.

E Carefully explain the risks and benefits of having a CT scan, looking up information first if you are uncertain.

F Tell her that she cannot have an MRI and clearly document that she refused the CT scan.

G Ask your consultant to visit on his ward round the following week to discuss management options.

H Use this question to identify a gap in your knowledge and read around the subject during a spare moment.

18. Your registrar suggests one morning before the ward round that your appearance is inappropriate. In particular, he says that you are showing too much of your chest and are wearing a watch.

Choose the THREE most appropriate actions to take in this situation

A Remove the watch immediately as it conflicts with Trust policy.

B Explain that you had not realized that your dress was inappropriate and will consider this before coming to work the next day.

C Point out that your consultant also wears a watch.

D Wear more revealing clothes the following day to show you are free to interpret the Trust dress code yourself.

E Tell your registrar that he should be more interested in your clinical ability than your choice of clothes.

F Decline to participate in the ward round because you have been insulted by the registrar.

G Tell your consultant that your registrar was insulting and bullying before the ward round.

H Seek feedback from other colleagues if you are uncertain whether your clothes really are inappropriate.

19. You are on call at night and have not eaten since coming to work. You are very tired and can feel yourself nodding off to sleep within a few seconds of sitting down. You are about to break away for a sandwich when a Ward Sister asks you to write two drug charts for patients who have just been admitted.

Choose the THREE most appropriate actions to take in this situation

A Explain that you were planning to go for a break.

B Offer to write the drug charts later on.

C Explain that writing drug charts is not a job for the on-call doctor and is best left to the ordinary ward team instead.

D Have a quick look, prescribe any urgent drugs, and then go for your sandwich.

E Ask the nurse to complete the drug chart for you to sign when you get back.

F Ask how urgent the drugs are and use this information to prioritize the task.

G Tell the nurse that she should not bother you for such a routine task.

H Complete the drug charts as requested.

20. You know that you do not always communicate well when feeling stressed and want to avoid this impacting on your relationship with colleagues.

Choose the THREE most appropriate actions to take in this situation

A Use 'team assessment of behaviour' (TAB) rounds and informal feedback from colleagues to gauge your success at managing stress.

B Tell other team members early on that they should avoid making you stressed.

C Ask other FY1s on your team to be responsible for shared tasks to minimize your workload.

D Make sure that you always go home at five o'clock.

E Try to streamline your work effectively so that you are not left with lots of tasks to complete at the end of the day.

F Talk to senior colleagues early if you think that the workload is getting on top of you.

G Drink alcohol in the evenings to 'loosen up'.

H Ask Human Resources (HR) for time each week to attend yoga and relaxation classes.

21. As the on-call FY1, you should finish at 10 p.m. and then hand over to the night SHO. However, one particular SHO refuses to accept jobs which he feels should have been completed during your shift. As a result, you find yourself leaving at 1 a.m. whenever he is scheduled to work nights.

Rank in order the following actions in response to this situation
(1 = Most appropriate; 5 = Least appropriate)

A Document that the SHO refused to accept a handover and then go home.

B Stay late if necessary to ensure that patient safety is not compromised.

C Raise the issue with an appropriate person (e.g. Educational Supervisor or line manager) as a priority on the following day.

D Report the night SHO to the GMC.

E Explain that you have completed as many tasks as you were able and that he should assume responsibility for them at the end of your shift.

22. You are a surgical FY1 expected to be prepared in advance of the morning ward round at 7.30 a.m. Your Clinical Supervisor tells you from the outset that you must also attend the 8 p.m. evening ward round. These hours conflict with the 9 a.m. to 5 p.m. working pattern indicated by your contract.

Rank in order the following actions in response to this situation
(1 = Most appropriate; 5 = Least appropriate)

A Remind your consultant that you are contracted to work between 9 a.m. and 5 p.m.

B Slip off home for a few hours each day to remain compliant with the European Working Time Directive.

C Ignore your consultant's instructions and work from 9 a.m. to 5 p.m. as you are required to do.

D Accept that long hours are an inevitable part of any surgical post.

E Seek advice from your Educational Supervisor.

23. Your registrar calls you during the day and tells you that a patient's suprapubic catheter has fallen out and needs to be reinserted. You explain that you have never done this before, but he says that it is simple and that no one else is free to help until the operating list finishes eight hours later. He is insistent.

Rank in order the following actions in response to this situation
(1 = Most appropriate; 5 = Least appropriate)

A Politely explain that you cannot perform the procedure safely and will need supervision.

B Ask another doctor with relevant experience to assist.

C Read about the procedure before having a go.

D Do as you are told but document carefully that you were acting under your registrar's instructions.

E Refuse to help as you are inundated with other ward jobs.

24. An elderly patient with pneumonia is deteriorating despite antibiotic treatment. As the on-call medical FY1, you plan to discuss changing antibiotics with the duty consultant microbiologist. However, the nursing staff and patient's family are united in wanting treatment to be withdrawn to stop the patient from suffering. You seem to be alone in wanting to continue treating the patient aggressively.

Rank in order the following actions in response to this situation
(1 = Most appropriate; 5 = Least appropriate)

A Familiarize yourself carefully with the case and try to understand why the family and nursing staff want to withdraw treatment.

B Insist on continuing with your plan as you are ultimately responsible for the patient.

C Stop all active treatment to hasten the patient's death and so end her discomfort.

D Contact a senior doctor to ask for their decision.

E Tell the patient's family to think carefully about the options and that you will do as they want if all members agree.

25. You are on call and bleeped by a ward nurse about a bag of blood which was mistakenly taken out of the fridge. As it cannot now be returned, she asks you to prescribe it for the patient so that it is not 'wasted'. You are not intending to visit the ward for some time and the nurse sounds frustrated as the blood will be lost 30 minutes after removal from the refrigerator.

Rank in order the following actions in response to this situation
(1 = Most appropriate; 5 = Least appropriate)

A Go to the ward immediately to prescribe the blood.

B Tell her that you will not authorize a transfusion simply to avoid waste.

C Tell her that she should not have removed the bag unnecessarily and complete a clinical incident form after your shift.

D Encourage her to put the bag back in the refrigerator so that it can be returned to blood bank for other patients.

E Explain that transfusion carries significant risks and there is no benefit in transfusing a non-anaemic patient.

26. An experienced staff nurse asks you to sign a prescription for a sleeping tablet which she administered an hour ago. You decline as this does not seem to be correct, but the Ward Sister says you have to sign as this is how things have always worked in their unit.

Rank in order the following actions in response to this situation (1 = Most appropriate; 5 = Least appropriate)

A Sign the prescription retrospectively.

B Tell both nurses that only doctors have the required training to decide which drugs to prescribe.

C Check the drug details to ensure that there were no contraindications and that an appropriate dose was administered.

D Advise that a note should be made on the prescription chart and hospital notes to indicate the drug was administered.

E Explain that an authorized prescriber must agree before drugs are given in future.

27. You are an FY1 and part of the cardiac arrest team. On arriving at an arrest, you find that no one is managing the patient's airway despite a number of senior doctors being present. Other appropriate activities are ongoing.

Rank in order the following actions in response to this situation (1 = Most appropriate; 5 = Least appropriate)

A Stand back so that you do not distract the arrest team leader.

B Ask the team leader why no one is managing the airway.

C Move to the patient's head and use airway adjuncts as appropriate.

D Ask whether an anaesthetist is present and, if not, whether they are on their way.

E Help with chest compressions because these are easily within your comfort zone.

28. The on-call bleep is constantly going off and you have a number of jobs to prioritize. You need to determine which to attend to first and then in order of priority.

Rank in order the following actions in response to this situation
(1 = Most appropriate; 5 = Least appropriate)

A A 55-year-old man with central chest pain.

B An angry daughter who wants to discuss why her mother is developing bed sores and is threatening a formal complaint.

C A 40-year-old woman with metastatic cancer with bony pain needing analgesia review.

D A 24-year-old man after an elective orthopaedic operation who wants to go home but first needs a discharge summary and prescription.

E A 90-year-old woman with a pneumonia who is hypotensive and became unresponsive a few moments ago.

29. You are clerking patients in the Emergency Department. Your current patient is in police custody and, at the point of discharge, the accompanying officers ask you for a copy of the discharge summary. The patient asks you not to provide them with any details but the officers insist that you *must* cooperate with their request.

Rank in order the following actions in response to this situation
(1 = Most appropriate; 5 = Least appropriate)

A Politely explain to the police officers that you cannot provide information without your patient's consent.

B Discuss with a consultant if the officers insist.

C Give a discharge summary to the patient knowing that it might be confiscated later on.

D Give the officers a discharge summary as helping the police is in the public interest.

E Tell the officers that there are no circumstances under which you would betray your patient's confidence.

30. You are called from the private wing of your hospital. The receptionist there asks for a cannula to continue a blood transfusion which is half completed. She called the responsible consultant at home who told her to bleep on the on-call FY1 to re-site the cannula.

Rank in order the following actions in response to this situation (1 = Most appropriate; 5 = Least appropriate)

A Decline to re-site the cannula and suggest that the consultant comes in from home to do so as it his private patient.

B Assess the urgency of the transfusion and prioritize according to your other tasks.

C Help if you are able but let the receptionist know that they should have someone capable of cannulating patients on site.

D Cannulate the patient but leave an invoice with the receptionist for £80.

E Contact a responsible person (e.g. duty manager) to ask about the appropriateness of attending to tasks in the private wing.

31. You are on call and are approached by a staff nurse who admits to giving an unfamiliar drug stat instead of as an infusion over 12 hours. She asks you to see the patient but not to tell anyone about the error.

Choose the THREE most appropriate actions to take in this situation

A Review the patient as a priority.

B Call the duty manager immediately to request that the nurse be removed from work.

C Explain that you cannot cover up the error but that you will let her speak with the Ward Sister first.

D See the patient but do not write in the notes to avoid causing the nurse career difficulties.

E Complete a formal incident form as soon as possible after the event.

F Call the intensive care registrar to discuss urgent transfer as the patient has been overdosed.

G Encourage the patient to vomit and prescribe intravenous fluids to flush out the drug.

H Tell the nurse that you cannot help but to bleep you if the patient deteriorates.

32. The daughter of an elderly patient asks you for an update about her mother's condition. A recent CT scan was suspicious of lung cancer and your patient has asked you not to tell anyone else to stop them worrying. The daughter says she 'knows something is wrong' and it is unfair to keep the family 'in the dark'.

Choose the THREE most appropriate actions to take in this situation

A Empathize with the daughter but explain that you cannot disclose this information without her mother's consent.

B Advise her you will call security if she persists in bothering you for information.

C Tell her that the CT was normal and that her mother will be discharged soon.

D Explain that her mother has asked you not to discuss certain aspects of her care with anyone.

E Tell her the results of the CT scan but ask her not to tell the patient that you have done so.

F Discuss with your patient at the next opportunity to ensure that she understands the effect that withholding information might have on close family members.

G Talk openly with the daughter as her mother is elderly and probably lacks capacity.

H Give her your consultant's mobile number so that she can discuss directly with your senior.

33. You are on call for medicine but are making no progress with your tasks because you are fielding so many bleeps. There are a number of acutely unwell patients on the wards awaiting assessment and the Emergency Department is now calling to inform you that patients are breaching.

Choose the THREE most appropriate actions to take in this situation

A Remove the batteries from your bleep and begin your existing tasks.

B Call your senior to let them know that you are not coping with the workload.

C Make a clear list of tasks in order of clinical priority.

D Explain to the Emergency Department that you have yet to assess potentially unwell patients and cannot assist for some time.

E Go to the Emergency Department but document that this distracted you from other tasks in case anything goes wrong.

F Have a coffee break now as you work better when rested and are unlikely to get lunch later.

G Draft a letter to the Chief Executive complaining about the effect of your workload on patient care.

H Tell the Emergency Department that the Trust should appoint more doctors if it wants to avoid patient breaches.

34. You are experiencing relationship difficulties at home and this is affecting your ability to cope at work. The radiologist has just refused a CT request which your consultant said is very urgent and you burst into tears after leaving the radiology department.

Choose the THREE most appropriate actions to take in this situation

A Take a few minutes to compose yourself, and then alert your consultant to the radiology decision.

B Send an email to your team explaining that you are very stressed and should be spared difficult tasks for the foreseeable future.

C Take a break and speak to a supportive colleague if possible.

D Go back and plead with the radiologist to accept your request.

E Contact the Medical Director to complain that the radiologist was obstructive.

F Tell Medical Staffing that you are unwell and have to go home to manage your domestic affairs.

G Ask another FY1 colleague to speak to the radiologist about your urgent CT request.

H Seek advice from your Educational Supervisor and/or Occupational Health if you continue to struggle at work.

35. You are a surgical house officer. The other FY1 on your firm has called in sick and you feel that the workload is unmanageable for a single person. Your SHO apologizes for leaving you with so much to do but says that he 'has to go to theatre' or his logbook will suffer.

Choose the THREE most appropriate actions to take in this situation

A Tell the SHO that patient care should come before his logbook.

B Explain to the SHO that you cannot cope and need some help.

C Explain to the senior nurse on each ward that they should not bleep you unless patients are 'really sick'.

D Tell the SHO that you would like to go to theatre instead as he will be more efficient on the ward anyway.

E Ensure that your consultant or another senior doctor on the team knows that you are working alone.

F Call in sick tomorrow in case your colleague is away again and you are left alone for a second day.

G Carefully prioritize jobs and explain to the senior nurse on each ward that you are working alone and might be slower to respond than usual.

H Delay all patient discharges until the following day when your colleague might have returned.

36. You are ambushed leaving the ward by a group of relatives who are angry about the care of one of your patients who is now on ITU. They are asking lots of questions and one is videoing the interaction using a smart phone.

Choose the THREE most appropriate actions to take in this situation

A Say 'no comment' and block the camera with your hand.

B Try to ignore the camera and act as you would if it was not there.

C Explain that you are unable to talk about a patient's care without their permission.

D Tell the relatives that the Ward Sister is in a better position to answer their questions.

E Contact security if you feel threatened or their presence is obstructing your work.

F Answer questions to defuse the situation.

G Tell the group that you are from another team and have never heard of this particular patient.

H Try to confiscate the camera as you do not wish to be videoed.

37. You did not complete any alcohol screening questionnaires for patients admitted the previous week. A senior doctor tells you that this means that the Trust will lose a lot of money and that you should 'make up' answers to the questions retrospectively. You seek support from your consultant who tells you to do it to keep the Trust happy.

Choose the THREE most appropriate actions to take in this situation

A Decline to complete screening questionnaires dishonestly.

B Complete the questionnaires as you have been told to do so by two senior colleagues.

C Contact a tabloid newspaper to report that Trusts are submitting false data for financial reward.

D Don't complete the questionnaires but tell the senior doctor that you did so.

E Explain that you will make a particular effort to complete screening questionnaires the following week if these are important for the Trust.

F Refuse to complete the questionnaires as they are unhelpful and interfere with patient care.

G Put the afternoon aside to call all discharged patients and complete the questionnaires by telephone interview.

H Explain that you realize the importance of the questionnaires to the Trust but that you do not think it is correct to complete the forms retrospectively.

38. A young patient with a pericardial effusion wants to leave hospital to attend his brother's wedding. Both the patient and his family plead with you to discharge him earlier than your consultant had initially planned, albeit without knowing his social circumstances. The patient appears to be very well and has normal observations.

Choose the THREE most appropriate actions to take in this situation

A Explain the risks of premature discharge, looking these up or seeking senior advice if you are uncertain.

B Tell the patient that your consultant's word is final and that he cannot leave earlier.

C Explain that the patient can self-discharge at any point if he wishes to do so.

D As the patient is haemodynamically stable, agree to discharging him earlier than planned.

E As the patient is haemodynamically stable, let him leave hospital for 24 hours to attend the wedding.

F Tell the patient that you won't stop him if he wants to go and that he can find the risks of pericardial effusion easily enough online.

G Tell your patient that his health should always come ahead of family engagements.

H Contact a senior doctor for advice.

39. You have finished a night shift and are exhausted. As you are preparing to go home, you receive a call from the day FY1 to say they are suffering from diarrhoea and vomiting and cannot work as a consequence. You are due to work the following night as well.

Choose the THREE most appropriate actions to take in this situation

A Tell the FY1 to pull himself together and come into work.

B Leave your bleep in a designated place.

C Let the site manager know that the day FY1 is unable to come to the hospital.

D Head home as you have already worked a full night shift and are unsafe to continue.

E Work as much of the day shift as you can before you cannot continue and need to alert the responsible manager.

F Continue working to the best of your ability.

G Keep holding the bleep but decline to review patients as you are tired and unsafe.

H Ask the responsible manager to arrange appropriate cover so you have time for sufficient sleep before returning to work.

40. An elderly patient with known dementia is attempting to leave the ward. He has punched a healthcare assistant who tried to encourage him back to his bay. You do not believe that he has capacity to leave the ward.

Choose the THREE most appropriate actions to take in this situation

A Try to talk to the patient from a safe distance.

B Tackle the patient's legs and try to break his fall.

C Contact security urgently.

D Try to conduct an Abbreviated Mental State Examination (AMTS) from a safe distance.

E Attend to the healthcare assistant's injuries as soon as it is appropriate to do so.

F Shout and wave at the patient to encourage him back into the ward.

G Sedate the patient with propofol for his own safety and the safety of others.

H Continue with your work as agitated patients are a problem for the nursing team.

ANSWERS

1. **C, D, E, B, A**

GMC guidance states that the doctor providing treatment (i.e. the operation in this example) is responsible for obtaining informed consent. He
can delegate this responsibility to someone who is suitably trained and
has sufficient knowledge about the operation and its risks. As an FY1,
you are unlikely to satisfy these criteria. Therefore the best option is
to explain your position to the registrar (C). He should then consent
the patient himself or delegate the responsibility to someone else. You
should not consent the patient (A).

You could potentially ask an appropriately qualified doctor from another
team to help (D). This is not the preferred option as such a person will
have other duties, may not know the patient, and is unlikely to be part
of the operating team. If ever in doubt, it is advisable to ask colleagues
for advice. Although you should ideally ask a senior doctor, experienced
nurses may also point out that you should not consent patients for complicated procedures in FY1 (E). Deferring the issue until later (B) risks
causing the patient's case to be cancelled.

2. **B, E, C, A, D**

Your priority in this case must be the safety of your patient, i.e. ideally
you should not perform a procedure with which you are unconfident.
However, it is also important that you learn practical procedures so that
you can be a full member of the team and avoid unnecessarily burdening
colleagues in future. In this case, a confident fellow FY1 may be the most
appropriate person to assist (B) with a relatively simple procedure.

If the ABG is urgent and you are inexperienced but understand how it
is performed, you could attempt the procedure before asking for help
(E). All doctors have varying degrees of experience and need practice to
improve. Although there is no absolute requirement to inform patients
how many times you have performed a procedure before, you should aim
to be upfront and honest. If there is a realistic chance of failing the ABG
due to inexperience, it would be polite to inform the patient first (C) if
this would not cause them undue anxiety.

If the duty medical registrar is free to supervise your ABG, this could
satisfy everyone (A). However, they are likely to have many demands on
their time and other options should be explored before interrupting their
other duties. Handing over an ABG because you are unconfident (D) is
the least helpful option. This is because the investigation has been delayed
unnecessarily, a colleague has been burdened with an additional task, and
your skills have not improved.

3. **B, D, A, C, E**

Your first priority in any patient about whom you are worried is to familiarize yourself with their details and ensure that they are stable (e.g.

Airway, Breathing, Circulation) (B). You should use hospital guidelines (D) wherever possible to educate yourself about the proper management of medical problems. Once you have seen the patient and tried to find the appropriate information yourself, you may wish to consult a senior doctor (A) for advice or to confirm that your own plan is correct.

Using unregulated online resources is commonplace but should be discouraged (C). Hospital guidelines, senior colleagues, and potentially authoritative books (e.g. *Oxford Handbook for the Foundation Programme*) are better sources of information.

Loop diuretics are not used to manage hypernatraemia, which you would soon find out if you consulted hospital guidelines or discussed with the medical registrar (E).

4. **A, D, B, C, E**

Doctors should understand (and be able to defend) any investigation or procedure they request. You should avoid taking responsibility for requests you do not understand, and it is particularly difficult to persuade a radiologist to accept a scan request that you do not understand yourself. Your best option is to ask the consultant (A) or another member of the team (D) what the scan is for.

Although the radiologist might understand why the scan is necessary (B), she cannot always be expected to know what your consultant was thinking. You should aim to be better informed than this before approaching a senior doctor outside of your team.

Your disagreement may be due to poor communication and/or your own misunderstanding rather than an inappropriate request. Aim to understand what your consultant is trying to achieve rather than being confrontational (C).

If you have been asked to request a CT, you should generally not do something else simply based on your own initiative (E). Given that your consultant is considerably more experienced, ordering an ultrasound instead may both delay the definitive investigation and waste a valuable ultrasound scanning slot that could be used by someone else.

5. **D, E, B, A, C**

Thankfully, no harm came to this patient as the error was spotted by the pharmacist. The most important thing now is that both you and the organization learn from this incident. Your NHS e-portfolio has a reflection area which is well suited to this purpose (D). There is a wider concern raised about the safety of your working hours. This should be raised with your Educational Supervisor (E) and/or rota coordinator in case a pattern emerges.

Although you should accept personal responsibility for your prescription (A), you should take steps to communicate the factors which you think contributed to the error (B) in whatever way is necessary to effect appropriate organizational change.

You should never seek to cover up your mistakes or ask colleagues to do so for you (C). If the Matron feels that the error if sufficiently serious to raise with your Educational Supervisor, you should not interfere with this decision.

6. B, E, D, A, C

Patient safety is your priority and someone should follow up this test result immediately. The duty house officer is the most appropriate person to do so (B). Although revisiting the hospital (E) may be necessary, you should try to maintain a work–life balance provided that you are able to ensure patient safety through other means. It is important to avoid such errors in future (you may not remember next time) and a simple change of routine, such as checking blood results at a set time of day (D), may be sufficient.

Checking investigation results for an unwell patient the next day (A) leaves them at risk overnight, as does forgetting the issue altogether (C).

7. A, C, B, D, E

You should first seek to clarify what has prompted your colleague's concerns (A). There may be good explanations or she might have noticed something that you have yet to pick up on yourself.

If there are concerns about any aspect of your health, these are best discussed in the first instance with your GP (C). GMC guidance states that all doctors should be registered with a GP so that objective advice can be sought if necessary. Although you should avoid 'corridor consultations' with colleagues whenever possible, your Educational Supervisor (B) may be an additional source of advice and support. Your FY1 colleagues have much less formal responsibilty for your pastoral well-being (D). While you might wish to involve them at some point as friends, you should avoid approaching junior colleagues for an independent assessment or medical advice. You should avoid trying to assess or treat yourself (E) for any significant medical condition.

8. C, D, E, B, A

GMC guidance states you must always be honest and recognize the limitations of your knowledge. Your best option here is to tell the patient what you know and explain that it is the limit of your knowledge (C). However, you should do what you can to ensure that the patient's questions are answered, and this may involve a senior doctor (D). This also creates an opportunity for you to learn the answer and see it communicated to a patient. As this identifies a gap in your knowledge, it may signpost an area to study for your own development (E).

The fact that you are an FY1 does not preclude you from answering complicated questions (B). If you were confident in your knowledge of stomas, you could have answered this patient fully yourself.

Telling the patient that his colostomy will be reversed is an error if you are uncertain and/or do not know the precise plan in this case (A).

9. A, C, D, E, B

Your ALS course will have taught you to call for help early (A) and then resuscitate the patient using an Airway, Breathing, Circulation approach (C). Calling a senior doctor on her mobile phone (D) might bring help (if she is available), but probably not enough for a patient deteriorating so quickly.

Seeking telephone advice from a senior colleague might at least lead to her suggesting that you summon the resuscitation team. Opting to continue managing the patient until he deteriorates further (E) or using him as a practice case (B) would involve working outside your ability as a single FY1 doctor.

10. A, C, D, E, B

If you genuinely think that the assessment is unfair, you should be upfront with a view to seeking further information (A). Whether or not you ultimately agree, this is clearly the impression with which your consultant has been left. Therefore you should ask her advice about how to improve (C), although clarifying the source of the concerns would be the most appropriate first step in this scenario. An e-portfolio TAB round might be useful to see how you come across to a broader selection of colleagues (D). If no one else expresses concerns, this might reassure both you and your consultant.

Individuals are often neither the most effective nor convincing judges of their own level of knowledge. Medical school performance may not indicate the type of knowledge needed as a doctor (E) and could give the impression that you are arrogant and/or lacking in insight. This option is best avoided.

It is difficult to claim a relationship breakdown based on a single episode of negative feedback (B). Only if a pattern of problems arose should you consider discussing with the Foundation Programme lead at your hospital.

11. D, E, G

All doctors should be registered with a GP whom they should approach with concerns about their health (D). Although there is no obligation to speak with your Educational Supervisor (E) if work is unaffected, they may be better placed to support you if they are kept informed. If your alcohol consumption has increased recently, you might wish to try reducing it for health and social reasons (G).

You should not threaten your physical health by attempting to provoke withdrawal symptoms (F). Although asking someone else for objective advice (A) on your drinking may be commendable, a social friend may not be the most appropriate person. You are already concerned about your drinking and should seek advice from an independent professional rather than attempting to manage the problem further yourself (C). Although you might be concerned about acquiring an unhelpful reputation, asking your colleagues to stop gossiping (B) may be ineffective and will not solve any underlying drinking problem. Drinking secretly will certainly not solve any such alcohol dependency (H).

12. B, C, F

Competence in intravenous cannulation is a fundamental skill for doctors and mandatory for successful completion of Foundation Year 1.

You should identify what exactly it is you find difficult about cannulation (B), ask for supervision and feedback (C), and then seek opportunities to improve your ability (F).

Strategies to avoid cannulating patients, such as asking colleagues to do it (A), avoiding 'difficult' cases (D), or calling a specialist after a token attempt (G), will burden others and will not help you to improve your ability. Covering your own deficiencies by blaming patients (H) is not encouraged, although it might be fair to warn patients if you genuinely anticipate that multiple attempts may be necessary.

Career aspirations could be modified if you find yourself struggling (and/ or not enjoying) practical procedures (E). However, it would be premature to make such decisions based on experiencing difficulties with one skill over such a short space of time.

13. C, G, H

GMC guidelines require all doctors to recognize the limits of their knowledge and experience. In this case, you have attempted to fluid resuscitate the patient without success. The next step is to seek advice and/or assistance from a senior colleague (C).

As a foundation doctor, you must be able to manage patients who are potentially deteriorating until help arrives. In this case, you should ensure that there is good intravenous access (G) and that the patient is being observed carefully (H) while you are waiting for support.

Although the patient's blood pressure may be acceptable for them, this should not be assumed without further information (B). Similarly, it is far from clear that the patient is peri-arrest (D), dying (F), or appropriate for a 'Not For Resuscitation' decision (A). Inotropes would not be an appropriate next step in this case (E).

14. A, B, E

It is important to remain professional at all times and to take necessary steps to avoid your own feelings affecting how you behave towards others. In this case, you should recognize early on that you are behaving unprofessionally and take remedial action. It may be helpful to take a short break (A), ask a colleague for assistance (B), and address any specific factors that you think may have contributed to your behaviour (E).

Although patients should always be your priority, dealing with relatives is an important job for junior doctors, even when on call (C). Apologizing to these particular relatives (D) may well be appropriate but the motivation for doing so should not be to avoid complaints. Clock watching is not a strong solution to the problem (H).

Action to remove relatives (F) should only be initiated if staff, patients, or other visitors are at risk. You should have sufficient insight to wonder whether two 'clashes' with relatives in quick succession may reflect your behaviour as much as theirs. The medical student (G) is not to blame!

15. C, D, G

You must comply as far as possible with any complaints procedure. In this case, you should cooperate with your line manager by providing factual details in a timely manner (C).

Regardless of the complaints process (and outcome), you must endeavour to improve your own practice. You may identify areas of clinical practice or communication which could be improved from this experience (D). As well as documenting carefully, you should ask for the complaint outcome (G) as to aid the learning process.

At all times you must be honest and trustworthy. GMC and local disciplinary procedures will expect this from all clinical staff. You must not edit the notes retrospectively to protect yourself (A) (B) or obstruct the process by not replying (E) or delaying your response (H).

Although you may need to explain your actions, being 'busy' is not an excuse for failing to examine a patient thoroughly (F). Doctors must take personal responsibility for their actions, even if other factors contribute.

16. B, E, F

As a junior doctor, you must recognize your own limitations at all times. In this case, you are uncomfortable with the request and must ensure patient safety even at the expense of upsetting your consultant.

You should be honest and communicate to the consultant that you are unhappy with his request (B). It may have been miscommunicated and/or your response may prompt the consultant to change his mind. If you feel pressured to work beyond your limitations, this should be raised with your Educational Supervisor at the first available opportunity (E). If you cannot re-contact the consultant, you should get in touch with another senior colleague (F) to discuss your concerns.

In this case, sedating a patient on a regular ward is likely to be unacceptable, even for a senior doctor (D). You must always prioritize patient safety over other considerations and should not comply with a request which you believe might be dangerous (A) (C) (H). Attempting to relocate the hip without sedation (G) would be very painful and may cause more harm if you are unfamiliar with the procedure.

17. D, E, H

You must always be open and honest about your knowledge. In this case, you should explain to the patient that you do not know the answer but endeavour to find out (D). This will also support your development. Once you have closed any gaps in your own knowledge (H), you should carefully explain the advantages and disadvantages of CT (E). *Good Medical Practice* states that this process is a necessary part of obtaining consent for any procedure or investigation.

You should not overburden senior colleagues (C) or delay an investigation (G) if you are able to answer a question adequately after looking up the answer. This risks distracting them from their own responsibilities. You can answer any question as long as it is within your knowledge and experience to do so adequately (B).

Making up an answer (A) is dishonest unless you know it to be true. Risks, benefits, and likely consequences should be explained before a competent patient is deemed to have refused a procedure (F).

18. A, B, H

Wearing a watch conflicts with Department of Health policy on staff dress in clinical areas. Its removal is likely to be a reasonable request (A). You should try to accept negative feedback and use it to reflect on changes you might make in future (B). If you disagree with negative feedback, you may wish to seek other views in a genuine attempt to improve your professional appearance (H).

You may wish to raise your consultant's compliance with policy at another time (C). However, this is not an adequate defence of your own behaviour and should not be raised with another colleague in this forum. You should not provoke your registrar or act in any way which makes him feel less able to give you feedback in future (D) (E) (F).

Although bullying is an important issue for doctors, this should be distinguished from a single episode of negative feedback (G).

19. A, B, F

Once again, patient safety must be your first consideration. Prescribing whilst stressed, hungry, and tired is more likely to lead to errors. You must balance the risk of a prescribing error against the risk of the drug chart being delayed (F).

A single task could be done quickly before getting rest. Two drug charts may take some time and therefore you could explain your position (A) and say that you will write them later on (B).

Drug charts must sometimes be written by the on-call medical team (C) (G) as drugs cannot be given without them. However, they are a source of prescribing errors as the on-call doctor is tired, balancing multiple tasks, and may not know the patient. Prescribing should be taken seriously and not done 'quickly' before going for a break (D). Ideally, drug charts should not be written by someone who is so tired that they are nodding off to sleep (H) or who is not an authorized prescriber (E).

20. **A, E, F**

Doctors must be familiar with their own strengths and weaknesses. The Foundation Programme e-portfolio has a number of tools (e.g. Team Assessment of Behaviour (TAB)) for reflecting on and so mitigating potential weaknesses (A). Effective time management can reduce stress levels (E), as can involving senior colleagues if work levels become unmanageable (F). Although you should always aim to leave on time, this will not always be possible and doctors must be prepared to show some flexibility (D) to ensure that patients and colleagues do not come to harm.

Increasing the burden on other junior colleagues (B) (C) is unlikely to be a successful long-term strategy. Although outside interests are important, drinking excessively (G) is unhelpful and HR is unlikely to agree to time away for yoga classes. (H).

21. **E, B, C, D, A**

You are entitled to go home at the end of a shift. Your rota is designed to create sufficient rest so that it is within the law and guarantees patient safety. In this situation, you should politely but firmly explain that you have done what you can and are now handing over remaining jobs (E). If this is unsuccessful, you must guarantee patient safety, even if this means staying late (B). However, the SHO's behaviour is unacceptable and cannot be allowed to continue as it compromises the well-being of colleagues and potentially patients as well. Therefore inform you should an appropriate person as soon as possible (C). Although unacceptable, the SHO's obstructive attitude is unlikely in itself to warrant referral to the GMC (D). Going home without handing over important tasks (A) puts patients at risk and jeopardizes continuity of care, which must be prioritized.

22. **A, E, D, C, B**

Doctors must sometimes work flexibly because of the unpredictable nature of their profession. However, your regular work pattern is a contractual right. Working outside these hours might conflict with the European Working Time Directive and should potentially increase your banding supplement. In the first instance, you should raise this issue politely with your Clinical Supervisor (A). If the response is unsatisfactory, your next source of help is your Educational Supervisor (E). Long hours can be imposed by your employer (within legal limits) but should be appropriately recognized and compensated. Working beyond your contracted hours (D) can risk your well-being and that of patients. Ignoring your Clinical Supervisor's expectations (C) is unprofessional and may create unnecessary conflict. Leaving the hospital without permission and arranging appropriate cover is unacceptable as important tasks (e.g. patients becoming unwell) may arise during working hours (B).

23. **A, B, C, D, E**

No doctor should work beyond their limitations. You should be very clear when letting seniors know that you are out of your depth (A). If there is genuinely no one from your team available, you should ask another senior colleague (e.g. the on-call surgeon) to perform or supervise the procedure (B). You should certainly exploit this learning opportunity (C), but only attempt a procedure if you are competent to do so. Documentation is important (D) but will not absolve you of responsibility if you perform a task inappropriately and the patient comes to harm as a consequence. FY1 doctors must prioritize tasks, and helping a patient who cannot pass urine should come before most routine ward tasks (E).

24. A, D, B, E, C

Ideally, grave decisions of this nature should be based on a broad consensus including doctors, members of the multi-disciplinary team, relatives, and the patient herself if possible. Therefore you should try to understand (and empathize with) opinions that conflict with your own (A). In general, FY1 doctors should not make end-of-life decisions and senior advice should be sought (D), particularly when there is no consensus (B). Although it is important to be open and negotiate, the medical team's prerogative should never be delegated in its entirety to third parties such as family members (E). Intentionally hastening death is murder under UK law, even if your motive is to end discomfort (C). Treatment can only be withdrawn if it is futile or your intention is to relieve specific suffering (e.g. high flow oxygen causing mucosal dryness, or intravenous fluids worsening pulmonary oedema).

25. E, B, C, A, D

Blood transfusion carries significant risks (including death) and should not be considered without good reason. This should be explained politely (E) rather than simply dismissing the nurse's request (B). Although the bag should not have been removed unnecessarily, in this case might uninvited criticism not be well received (C). The blood should not be administered to the patient without good reason (A) under any circumstances as this exposes them to unnecessary risk. You should not tamper with blood products or encourage anyone else to do so (D) as this risks the health of whichever patient ultimately receives the blood.

26. C, D, E, A, B

Patient safety must be your first priority. Therefore you should ensure that the drug and dose given have not exposed the patient to risk (C). Whether or not the drug is prescribed retrospectively, a note must be made on the drug chart (D) so that a clear record exists that it has been administered. Even if this has become common practice on the unit, only an authorized prescriber should approve drugs to be administered (E). Once the other issues have been addressed, you may choose whether or not to accept responsibility by signing retrospectively (A). You are not obliged to prescribe the drug simply because it was given. It would be incorrect and unhelpful to say that only doctors can prescribe (B) as many other healthcare professionals can prescribe under certain circumstances (e.g. nurse-prescribers).

27. **C, D, B, E, A**

Maintenance of the airway must be prioritized in an arrest situation. If no one is managing the airway and you are comfortable doing so with basic adjuncts, you should take responsibility for this task (C). However, you will need senior support, so seek the presence of an anaesthetist (D). Although the team leader has many distractions, you must raise your concern if the airway is not being managed by you or anyone else (B). Although chest compressions are an important task and must continue, you should not ignore an airway concern simply to remain within your comfort zone (E). You have a duty to help if there is an opportunity to do so and should raise your concern as a minimum (A).

28. **E, A, C, B, D**

A critically ill patient who is deteriorating and may be peri-arrest should be your priority (E) regardless of her age. The patient with central chest pain should be reviewed early as he could become unstable (A). Severe pain should be treated as an emergency (C) for compassionate reasons—patients should not be left in pain when relief is available. Although urgent, the angry relative's demand must be secondary to the immediate requirements of other patients (B). However, bed sores are a serious concern and you should try to discuss this situation to improve her mother's care and avert a complaint if possible. Therefore this situation should be prioritized above the young patient awaiting discharge (D), however keen he is to go home.

29. **A, B, C, E, D**

You must respect patient confidentiality whenever possible and explain this politely (A). However, if the police officers are insistent, you might wish to check with a senior that guidance has not changed (B). It may be appropriate to give the patient a copy of his discharge summary (C), but not if this is a masked attempt to provide one to the officers.

It is incorrect to say that there are no circumstances under which confidentiality would be breached (E). For example, this may be possible to avert a serious crime and limited cooperation is possible in specific cases (e.g. firearms offences). Nevertheless, you should not decide yourself to provide a discharge summary to the police when your patient has clearly refused consent (D).

30. **B, C, E, A, D**

Covering the private wing might not be one of your usual responsibilities. However, you may have a duty to help a patient in extremis (e.g. Hb 5.0 and mid-way through a transfusion) (B). Although you should help if possible, the private wing should not depend on NHS resources unless this has been agreed with your Trust (C). You might wish to check with an appropriate person about attending to tasks in the private wing, particularly if they are non-urgent (E). If the task is not an emergency, you may decline to help on principle or if other jobs take priority. However, the consultant may not be able to reach the hospital in time to save the unit of blood being wasted (A). If you agree to help, you should not attempt to charge the private wing (D), particularly while you are already being paid to work by your NHS employer.

31. **A, C, E**

This patient has had an accidental overdose and needs to be reviewed as a priority (A). You must not wait until the patient shows signs of deterioration (H). Although you must not cover up clinical errors (D), the nurse may prefer to inform the Ward Sister herself (C). As this is a serious error, a formal incident report must be completed contemporaneously (E) so that a paper trail is created and lessons can be learned. There is no need to think that this nurse is an immediate danger to other patients (B). It would be inappropriate to discuss with intensive care (F) until you have assessed the patient and have decided that higher-level care is necessary. Intravenous fluids and vomiting are not standard interventions (G) and would only be indicated on senior advice or if directed by a reliable resource (e.g. Toxbase).

32. **A, D, F**

You should be sensitive to the daughter's concern but firm that you cannot breach confidentiality in this case (A). You may indicate that you have not been given permission to give details to anyone (D). It might be helpful to let your patient know that close family members are anxious for details (F) in case she changes her mind and agrees to involve them. Calling security (B) is an overreaction and likely to inflame the situation. You must not lie (C) or breach your patient's confidentiality (E), even if you feel coerced by her family. Capacity is not age-dependent (G) and cannot be assumed to be lacking in an elderly patient. Your consultant is unlikely to approve of his contact details being given out (H)—colleagues are also entitled to a degree of confidentiality.

33. **B, C, D**

You have a duty to speak out whenever you feel that patient care is being compromised. In this case you should let a senior know (B) if you are unable to cope—they might be able to help or redirect resources accordingly. A clear jobs list will help you prioritize tasks so that the most urgent are completed first (C). You must not neglect potentially unwell patients to meet other commitments (e.g. hospital targets) (D), even if you document the reason (E). However, you should not be discourteous or facetious when declining to help the Emergency Department (H) to maintain good working relations. Time spent on a coffee break (F) or drafting a letter (G) could be better used to assess your potentially unwell patients. You should never render yourself uncontactable (A) in case emergencies require your immediate attention.

34. **A, C, H**

If the CT request is very urgent, you should alert your consultant (A) if there is any reason why it cannot go ahead. You might have miscommunicated its urgency and/or he might want to intervene. You should take some time to compose yourself and speak to a supportive colleague if one is available (C). If you are finding things particularly difficult, you should seek independent advice from your GP, Educational Supervisor, and/or Occupational Health (H). Talking again to the radiologist (D) or asking a colleague to do so (G) is unlikely to be helpful unless the situation has changed or more facts are available.

The radiologist may have good reason to decline your request and is not necessarily being obstructive (E). In any event, the Medical Director would not be your first port of call. You should only ask to go home (F) if you cannot continue working, as this may disrupt patient care and is unlikely to resolve your difficulties. A generic email asking others to shoulder your work (B) might be misinterpreted and/or unfairly burden colleagues.

35. B, E, G

You should not accept a situation which compromises patient care and your first action should be to reason with the SHO (B). This should be done in a non-confrontational manner (A). If you cannot source additional support, you must let a senior member of the team know that you are under-staffed on the ward (E). You should let nursing colleagues know in advance that you might be slower to respond than usual (G). However, you should never discourage staff from calling you about deteriorating patients (C)—more can be done for unwell patients who are identified early.

If the ward team is short-staffed, you should not seek to leave your SHO alone to cope (D). The SHO might be a surgical trainee who will learn more (and be more useful) in theatre than an FY1. You must not fake illness (F) as this is dishonest and unfair to colleagues who will be even more stretched the following day. Patient discharges should not be delayed unnecessarily (H) but might be lower priority than some tasks.

36. B, C, E

FY1 doctors must remain resilient under pressure. In this case, you should try to ignore the camera (B) and act normally by explaining politely that you cannot discuss a patient's case without their permission (C). Do not breach confidentiality simply because the situation is pressurized (F). You have a right not to feel threatened at work and should call security for assistance if you feel out of your depth (E). Trying to obscure (A) or confiscate (H) the camera will aggravate the situation and look very bad on tape afterwards! You should not lie under any circumstances (G) but politely decline to answer questions. Although directing relatives to the correct member of staff (D) might be helpful, the result in this case would simply be to shift an uncomfortable situation onto a nursing colleague.

37. A, E, H

There are very few circumstances which justify dishonesty and this is not one of them. You should not complete the questionnaires with false data (A) (B).

However, you should recognize your omission and let your senior know your plan to improve the following week (E). Empathizing with the senior doctor and demonstrating that you understand their importance (H) will help defuse any potential conflict. Refusing outright to participate (F) is likely to result in conflict and is at odds with your status as a Trust employee. However, the questionnaires need to be prioritized alongside other tasks and an afternoon calling patients for this purpose is poor use of clinical time (G). Lying to a senior doctor, even if this might appear to solve the problem, is unjustifiable and could result in professional difficulties (D). Raising concerns with a newspaper in the first instance would be likely to result in employment and/or professional disciplinary action (C)

38. A, C, H

You cannot prevent a patient with capacity from leaving hospital and the patient should be aware that he is free to leave at any time (C) (B). However, you have a duty to ensure that he understands the associated risks and should find these out if you are unsure (A) (F). If you are concerned about the patient's decision, you might consult a senior (H) who could potentially counsel the patient more convincingly.

If your consultant has made a clinical plan, you should not contradict this without very good reason (D) (E). FY1 doctors must be open to patients having different values and life priorities. It is acceptable for a patient to prioritize a family engagement (G) as long as he understands the potential consequences of doing so.

39. C, F, H

Although, ideally, you should not work when exhausted, it would be more dangerous for you to leave without a replacement (D) or to become uncontactable (B). You should continue working (F) but let a manager know at the earliest opportunity so that relief can be sought (C) (E). As you are due to work the following night, the manager should arrange sufficient cover so that you are not still exhausted on returning to the hospital (H). You must continue to review patients who are potentially unwell, even if you are tired (G).

Your FY1 colleague should not come to work with diarrhoea and vomiting as there is a risk of spreading Norovirus to vulnerable patients (A).

40. A, C, E

Although the patient has dementia, you should first try to communicate him as with any patient (A). As he has already hit a healthcare assistant, he may continue to be violent and need to be restrained. Security officers are the most appropriate people for this task (C). Once the situation is controlled, you should attend to any injuries arising, including to staff (E). You should not do anything likely to scare the patient (F) or cause harm (B) and should treat him with as much dignity as the situation permits. An AMTS assessment is unlikely to be successful or add very much to his immediate management (D). FY1 doctors should not give anaesthetic drugs (G), let alone in an unmonitored ward environment—propofol is not a solution in this case.

An agitated patient risks harming themselves or others and therefore is the responsibility of all staff (H).

Effective communication

Introduction

Questions within this section assess your ability to communicate effectively with patients and colleagues. Effective communication requires understanding and being understood.

You will need to demonstrate an ability to negotiate with colleagues, to document information within the medical notes clearly and concisely, to gather information from patients, and to listen to angry relatives. As always, your responses must adapt to the needs and context of each situation, while always remembering to demonstrate empathy and compassion.

- Listen to patients, relatives, and colleagues. They are trying to tell you something.
- Explain your position carefully after listening to the other side.
- Adapt your style as far as possible to the person with whom you are communicating.
- However strongly you feel, poor manners will never get the job done faster.

QUESTIONS

1. You are covering medical wards at the weekend when you are asked by a nurse to speak to the relatives of a patient about his newly diagnosed malignancy. You have not met the patient before but are told that his relatives are very anxious.

Rank in order the following actions in response to this situation
(1 = Most appropriate; 5 = Least appropriate)

A Establish how much the relatives wish to know, and respond to their requests honestly and with compassion.

B Politely decline to discuss the health of the patient without his explicit permission.

C Ask the nurse to read the medical notes and speak to the family after doing so.

D Explain that you do not know the patient and that they should speak to the regular ward team instead.

E Collectively address both the patient's and the family's concerns, and answer each of their questions in turn.

2. You have been shown how to insert chest drains and have been asked to do so for a patient on your ward. You intend to obtain consent but recall that this can be found to be invalid afterwards unless the patient is warned about important complications.

Rank in order the following actions in response to this situation
(1 = Most appropriate; 5 = Least appropriate)

A Ask the patient what risks of chest drain insertion he knows about.

B Obtain legal advice before consenting.

C Speak to the consultant prior to obtaining consent.

D Ensure accurate and complete documentation of the consent.

E Ask for a nurse to be present during the consent process.

3. You are working as an FY1 at night in the surgical assessment unit, when you are asked to clerk an elderly patient who is profoundly deaf and unable to write.

Rank in order the following actions in response to this situation
(1 = Most appropriate; 5 = Least appropriate)

A Attempt a brief verbal history.

B Skip the history, and focus your management on the examination and investigations.

C Do not attempt a history without a translator present.

D Complete your detailed history via handwritten questions.

E Extrapolate a history based on the limited findings of the ambulance crew on their initial assessment sheet.

4. Your next patient at the gynaecology clinic arrives with her brother-in-law, who explains that she is unable to speak any English. As you begin the interview you start to suspect that her brother-in-law is only communicating some of the information.

Rank in order the following actions in response to this situation
(1 = Most appropriate; 5 = Least appropriate)

A Reiterate to the brother-in-law that you need him to translate word for word.

B Try to establish whether the patient is happy with her brother-in-law acting as interpreter.

C Schedule another appointment with a formal interpreter.

D Invite the clinic receptionist into the consultation as she claims to speak a similar language to the patient's.

E Ask the brother-in-law to leave and complete the consultation without any interpreter.

5. You are on a busy orthopaedic ward round with your consultant when a nurse mentions that one of your patients drinks 60 units of alcohol per week. He is scheduled for an elective knee replacement in two days but is otherwise fit and healthy.

Choose the THREE most appropriate actions to take in this situation

A Ask the consultant to review the issue during the ward round.

B Return to the patient after the ward round to discuss the matter further with him.

C Prescribe pabrinex and chlordiazepoxide while the consultant consents the patient.

D Discuss the matter further with the patient during the ward round.

E Tell the patient to stop drinking alcohol.

F Mention the issue to the registrar after the ward round.

G Ask the nurse to keep superfluous information until after the ward round to avoid interruptions.

H Inform the drug and alcohol services representative.

6. A 50-year-old is admitted to hospital with a severe sudden-onset headache, which you think is probably a migraine. Your registrar asks you to telephone the on-call radiologist at home to authorize an urgent CT scan. You become distracted completing other jobs for the registrar and only remember to telephone the radiologist an hour later.

Rank in order the following actions in response to this situation
(1 = Most appropriate; 5 = Least appropriate)

A Inform the registrar about the delay, and phone the radiologist immediately to request the CT head scan.

B Phone the radiologist and explain that the registrar only just asked you to arrange the CT.

C Phone the radiologist and explain that the registrar wants the CT head scan but you think that it is likely to be a migraine.

D Ask the registrar to call the consultant radiologist himself.

E Phone your own consultant and ask for advice first.

7. At the end of your shift, you are told that a new patient has arrived under the care of your team. The nurse reads a long list of jobs which need completing and asks if you would address these before leaving. This is the third consecutive day that you will leave the ward late.

Rank in order the following actions in response to this situation (1 = Most appropriate; 5 = Least appropriate)

A Leave and review the jobs in the morning.

B Review the jobs and perform those which will take less than 15 minutes.

C Review the jobs that appear most urgent and complete these before handing over to the on-call doctor.

D Ask the nurses to contact the on-call doctor who can then review the patient.

E Ask the nurses to do what they can and to contact the on-call doctor if they feel that anything else must be done before the next morning.

8. You are the surgical FY1 on call, and are assessing an acutely unwell patient. This takes you until the end of your shift and leads to the accumulation of many ward jobs. The overnight surgical FY2 to whom you hand over is infuriated with your 'slow pace', and threatens to complain to your consultant in the morning unless you assist her.

Choose the THREE most appropriate actions to take in this situation

A Apologize for your failure to complete the ward jobs.

B Ask for feedback in order to improve your management and handover.

C Offer to continue working up the previously unwell patient who is now stabilized.

D Offer to assist with the ward jobs until she feels that the list of jobs has become more manageable.

E Do not hand her any more jobs, in an effort to avoid antagonizing her.

F Explain that you are unable to complete any more jobs now that your shift is over.

G Phone the surgical registrar in order to help resolve the apparent conflict.

H Complain to her consultant in the morning.

9. You are working on call as the medical FY1 when you are called to review a patient who has fallen. You stabilize the patient with ABCDE-directed management and complete a brief focused history and examination. You then make a telephone call to your registrar after planning first in your mind which details should be relayed.

Rank in order the following actions in response to this situation
(1 = Most appropriate; 5 = Least appropriate)

A May I speak with you about an 80-year-old patient, admitted with falls, who has fallen again this evening?

B The patient is now in atrial fibrillation, and I think that this may have contributed to her fall. Her past medical history is significant for stroke.

C My plan is to arrange an X-ray of her right hip and then speak to you about managing her new atrial fibrillation. What should I do next?

D Hello I am the medical FY1 on call.

E I have informed the consultant at home.

10. As the FY1 for a medical team, you are seeing a patient for the first time on the Monday ward round. You realize that the admitting doctors on Friday did not arrange a review by the weekend medical team, despite grossly abnormal blood results. What would you include as part of your written entry in the medical notes?

Choose the THREE most appropriate actions to take in this situation

A Your opinion as to whether it was appropriate to be reviewed by the weekend medical team.

B 'This patient was not seen by a weekend review team.'

C Include medical entries for the weekend by assessing the patient retrospectively.

D Both Friday's and Monday's blood results.

E Today's blood results only.

F Today's management plan.

G Avoid writing anything but review the patient.

H Tell the patient that the doctors treating him initially had done so incorrectly.

11. Your consultant asks you to insert a peripheral cannula into the vein of a large 14-year-old boy with learning difficulties. His parents are very anxious about the procedure after the distress caused during previous attempts at venepuncture. They ask whether a sedative could be used just before the procedure.

Choose the THREE most appropriate actions to take in this situation

A Trick the boy into having the cannula inserted by hiding the equipment from him until the last possible moment.

B Use a play therapist to familiarize the patient with the procedure, even though this might take several hours.

C Explain to the parents that you will insert the Venflon in the middle of the night when the patient is least likely to resist.

D Explain to the parents that it would be safer to physically restrain the child.

E Explore the anxieties of the parents before pursuing a mutually agreed plan.

F Offer to use an intramuscular sedative to 'help him sleep' during the procedure.

G Ask to cannulate the parents first in order to demonstrate the procedure to the patient.

H Talk to the patient to see how he would feel about the procedure.

12. You are involved in a clinical research project, taking consent for the collection of an additional oesophageal biopsy during oesophagogastroduodenoscopy (OGD). A patient with long-standing gastric reflux disease arrives for her regular OGD. She is very pleasant and accommodating, but is known to be anxious prior to OGD procedures.

Rank in order the following actions in response to this situation
(1 = Most appropriate; 5 = Least appropriate)

A As she is anxious and unlikely to want further information, briefly explain that she can help with medical research if she signs a consent form.

B Explain the complications from the OGD, and how one additional biopsy adds very little to her total risk from the procedure.

C Try to alleviate her future anxiety by explaining that she is participating in a trial which will eventually lead to the development of less invasive methods of oesophageal examination.

D Take the extra biopsy, but wait until after the procedure to obtain consent from the patient and before using any of the samples for research.

E Do not include the patient in the study, given her level of anxiety.

13. You are looking after several unwell patients as the medical FY1 covering wards at the weekend when a Sister asks you for an urgent discharge summary to help relieve a bed crisis in the hospital. She sympathizes with your workload but insists that a discharge letter must be written immediately.

Rank in order the following actions in response to this situation
(1 = Most appropriate; 5 = Least appropriate)

A Acknowledge the severity of the bed crisis, but refer her to your registrar, explaining that you have more urgent matters to attend to.

B Phone the registrar and ask if there are any spare junior doctors who can assist with your tasks.

C Offer to write the discharge letter once you have stabilized your patients.

D Ask the Ward Sister to complete the discharge letter but sign a blank copy in advance to expedite the discharge.

E Take two minutes to write a brief discharge letter before returning to the care of your patients.

14. A patient with newly diagnosed terminal lung cancer asks to see you on the general medicine ward. He would like to make a complaint about your registrar, whom he feels has failed to offer him treatment that might prolong his life.

Rank in order the following actions in response to this situation
(1 = Most appropriate; 5 = Least appropriate)

A Empathize with the patient's traumatic experience and offer to raise the matter with the registrar and consultant.

B Defend the registrar's actions, highlighting their knowledge and experience, and the generally poor prognosis of most lung cancers irrespective of the treatment modality.

C Explore the patient's concerns further.

D Inform the patient that you will refer him to the oncologist to consider chemo/radiotherapy.

E Offer him the services of an appropriate religious leader to address any spiritual questions he may have.

15. You are working in a team of three surgical FY1s. Tim, one of the surgical FY1s, routinely fails to complete his daily tasks despite leaving the ward on time every day. You decide to address the matter after leaving another shift more than an hour late in order to complete Tim's tasks.

Rank in order the following actions in response to this situation
(1 = Most appropriate; 5 = Least appropriate)

A Share any additional workload between yourself and the other surgical FY1 without involving Tim in the matter.

B Inform Tim of your additional workload and ask him whether he is experiencing any difficulties in completing his routine jobs.

C Speak to your other surgical FY1 colleague and encourage her not to complete Tim's routine tasks.

D Demand that Tim arranges a meeting with his foundation and clinical supervisors in order to 'address his failings'.

E Inform your consultant.

16. Phlebotomy rounds have been cancelled. You delegate venesection to your ward team. A nurse refuses to take blood from a patient who is being investigated for HIV.

Rank in order the following actions in response to this situation
(1 = Most appropriate; 5 = Least appropriate)

A Explain the ethical responsibility of medical staff to all patients.

B Demand that the nurse attempt to take the blood sample, or else she will be reported.

C Ask about her concerns about the task, and what could be done to improve her confidence in this situation.

D Take the sample yourself.

E Instruct another nurse to take the sample, but avoid telling them about the patient's possible HIV status to avoid frightening them.

17. You are preparing to finish your ward shift and must leave on time to catch a flight to the test centre, where you are due to sit an important examination. There are still two patients left to see as part of your ward round. Both are stable and awaiting input from social services, but your visit is likely to be prolonged by family members who are currently visiting.

Rank in order the following actions in response to this situation
(1 = Most appropriate; 5 = Least appropriate)

A Perform a quick examination of each patient without speaking to them or their families.

B See the patients but explain that you cannot spend much time with their relatives today, and that someone will be available to answer questions tomorrow.

C Ask the nurses to remove the families before briefly reviewing each patient.

D Assess the patients as usual and answer any questions the family members may have, even if this results in missing your flight.

E Explain to the nurses that the patients will be seen on tomorrow's ward round, and catch your flight.

18. You are interested in orthopaedic surgery and have been asked to 'scrub in' and assist with a total knee replacement. The orthopaedic surgeon is willing to spend longer with you in theatre provided that you consent the patient. You have not obtained consent for a surgical procedure before, but understand about some possible complications.

Rank in order the following actions in response to this situation
(1 = Most appropriate; 5 = Least appropriate)

A Admit to the patient that you are unfamiliar with consenting for the procedure but that he can ask the consultant later on if he has questions that you cannot answer.

B Attempt to consent the patient, and refer any specific questions to the anaesthetist who will conduct a preoperative assessment later on.

C Refuse to consent the patient.

D Ask the consultant to run through the procedure with you before consenting the patient.

E Ask the surgical registrar to consent the patient.

19. You are asked to speak to a new patient who is a suspected intravenous drug user and has been admitted recently following an opiate overdose. He has repeatedly been asked to stay in bed but continues to wander and demands to be allowed to leave.

Rank in order the following actions in response to this situation
(1 = Most appropriate; 5 = Least appropriate)

A Explain the nature of his admission and the dangers of discharge, and reiterate the risk of death if he were to self-discharge.

B Explore his reasons for wanting to self-discharge.

C Obtain the details of his family and ask them to get involved.

D Address any concerns or approaches adopted by the nursing staff which may be antagonizing the patient

E Do not attempt to engage with a person who has recently used intravenous drugs, as they are unlikely to be cooperative.

20. You have been asked to complete a death certificate for a patient whose care you were briefly involved in during the last few days of his life. There were no suspicious circumstances surrounding his death, but you are unclear about its precise cause. The mortuary staff suggest that you speak with someone else first if you are not sure.

Choose the THREE most appropriate actions to take in this situation

A Telephone your consultant.

B Telephone your registrar.

C Telephone the duty pathologist.

D Telephone the coroner's officer.

E Contact the ward clerk.

F Contact the nursing staff who looked after the patient.

G Telephone the patient's next of kin.

H Telephone the local police.

21. You are clerking a young child in A&E who has been admitted with suspected bronchiolitis. Physical examination is unremarkable except for a moderate wheeze, although you note that the parents appear somewhat unkempt, with dirty hands and clothes. You consider what to document as part of your findings in the medical notes.

Rank in order the following actions in response to this situation
(1 = Most appropriate; 5 = Least appropriate)

A Your opinion of the parent's treatment of the child, based on their appearance.

B Detailed physical examination and objective clinical assessment of the child.

C A brief summary of your clinical assessment.

D Complete your notes after they have been confirmed by a senior.

E Complete your notes later on after getting through a few more patients to keep the clinic moving.

22. You are working as the only junior doctor for the ortho-geriatric team, assessing a patient who has had a fall. You are bleeped by a nurse on another ward about one of your outliers who has become febrile. While you are taking this call, your crash bleep starts to sound.

Rank in order the following actions in response to this situation
(1 = Most appropriate; 5 = Least appropriate)

A Document your current assessment of the patient who has fallen and then attend your other commitments.

B Attend the crash call and then return to write in the notes retrospectively for the fallen patient.

C Attend the crash call and then see the pyrexial patient before documenting your assessment of the patient who fell.

D Avoid documenting the fallen patient as you are likely to be distracted by other tasks after attending the crash call and seeing the pyrexial patient.

E Allow other members of the crash team to attend the arrest while you complete all your documentation.

23. You are working alone in the afternoon on your colorectal ward as the FY1 being shadowed by a final-year medical student. The nurse informs you that a patient is looking increasingly unwell, a peripheral venous cannula needs siting for a blood transfusion, and another patient's family wishes to speak with you in private.

Choose the THREE most appropriate actions to take in this situation

A Assess the unwell patient alone.

B Assess the unwell patient with the medical student.

C Ask the medical student to assess the patient alone, and join him as soon as possible.

D Ask the student whether he wishes to try to place the peripheral venous cannula.

E Attempt to insert the peripheral venous cannula yourself.

F Speak to the patient's family with a nurse present.

G Speak alone to the patient's family.

H Ask the student whether he would be comfortable speaking to the family.

24. While you are working in A&E, a nurse informs you that a 33-week pregnant woman is being brought by helicopter into resuscitation following a road traffic collision. She asks you to prepare for her arrival in approximately five minutes. Your registrar has already been informed, and he asks you to call for assistance while he bleeps the obstetric team.

Choose the THREE most appropriate actions to take in this situation

A Inform the neonatal registrar.

B Call the orthopaedic consultant at home.

C Fast bleep the haematology registrar.

D Summon the cardiac arrest team.

E Request a phototherapy light.

F Call the switchboard and ask them to put out a trauma call.

G Ask a nurse to find a neonatal Resuscitaire and bring it to resuscitation.

H Ensure that there are medical students present to maximize the learning opportunity.

25. While working on call, you are asked to cannulate a large patient who requires intravenous antibiotics for a suspected diarrhoeal infection. Your bleep sounds for a third time during your fourth cannulation attempt when you finally believe that you have obtained access.

Rank in order the following actions in response to this situation
(1 = Most appropriate; 5 = Least appropriate)

A Stop your attempt immediately and answer your bleep.

B Secure and flush the cannula before answering your bleep.

C Try to get the attention of the Ward Sister so that she can answer your bleep.

D Answer your bleep after securing and flushing the cannula, cleaning the work area, and saying goodbye to the patient.

E Ignore the bleep as they will call again if it is important.

26. A patient on your ward is diagnosed with anal cancer. He tells you that his community would react very negatively if they knew of his diagnosis. As a result, he is very anxious that no one finds out, including his family.

Rank in order the following actions in response to this situation
(1 = Most appropriate; 5 = Least appropriate)

A Promise to remove any mention of anal cancer from his notes.

B Tell the patient that you will remove any mention of his diagnosis from patient lists.

C Tell the patient that his family are bound to find out at some point and it would be better if he told them.

D Let the nursing staff know that his family are not aware of the diagnosis.

E Treat him as any other patient under your care.

27. You hear Karen, one of the nurses, speaking unpleasantly to a child on the paediatric ward. The child is known to be particularly challenging to work with, and has a history of learning difficulties and behavioural problems.

Rank in order the following actions in response to this situation
(1 = Most appropriate; 5 = Least appropriate)

A Approach the pair, and ask to speak to Karen.

B Speak to a senior nurse before approaching Karen.

C Ask other staff working on the ward whether they have noticed any inappropriate behaviour recently.

D Do not raise any concerns as the child is not at risk.

E Inform the hospital Trust.

28. A patient who was admitted for an exacerbation of chronic obstructive pulmonary disorder (COPD) is upset about the standard of care she has received over the weekend. She would like to speak with you about the possibility of making a complaint.

Rank in order the following actions in response to this situation
(1 = Most appropriate; 5 = Least appropriate)

A Suggest that making a formal complaint is unlikely to resolve the situation.

B Provide contact details for the Patient Advice and Liaison Service (PALS) to see what they can offer.

C Discuss what happened over the weekend to upset her.

D Inform your consultant that the patient is considering making a complaint.

E Inform the patient that weekend medical cover is often inadequate and that a formal complaint might help to improve staffing levels.

29. You are being shadowed by a medical student during a long day in A&E. The student is very keen to help with procedures and you ask him to catherize Mr Wills. When you enter the room, the urinary catheter is partly inserted but you realize that you have directed the student to the wrong patient.

Choose the THREE most appropriate actions to take in this situation

A Ask the student to stop catheterizing the patient immediately.

B Write a clinical incident form.

C Tell the student that he should go home as he should have checked the patient's wristband.

D Allow the student to continue inserting the catheter in case it is necessary anyway.

E Allow the student to insert the catheter, but take it out afterwards before telling the patient it was to obtain a clean urine sample.

F Ask the student to apologize to Mr Wills.

G Accept full responsibility for the error.

H Obtain an ultrasound kidney–ureter–bladder (KUB).

30. Your registrar asks you to consent a patient whom you have clerked in A&E for a scrotal exploration with possible orchidopexy/orchidectomy. He is unable to consent the patient as he is in the emergency theatre with the patient already in the anaesthetic room.

Rank in order the following actions in response to this situation
(1 = Most appropriate; 5 = Least appropriate)

A Ask that he consent the patient with an 'acute scrotum' as soon as the emergency case is finished.

B Ask the registrar to contact the consultant at home.

C Phone the medical registrar on call.

D Attempt to take consent as well as you are able to.

E Ask a surgical SHO who has performed the operation in the past to take the consent.

31. You are asked to speak to a patient's relative who appears angry. He tells you outright that he is recording the conversation 'for legal purposes'. He has a number of questions, one of which is why his brother had a CT head instead of an MRI scan.

Choose the THREE most appropriate actions to take in this situation

A Say 'no comment' and refuse to speak until the tape recorder is turned off.

B Ignore the tape recorder and act as you would if it was not there.

C Explain that you are unable to answer his questions.

D Tell the relative that the Ward Sister is in a better position to answer his questions.

E Contact security if you feel threatened or his presence is obstructing your work.

F Answer his questions politely.

G Tell the man that you are from another team and have never heard of this particular patient.

H Try to turn off the tape recorder yourself.

32. You have arranged a bedside teaching session using a patient with known inoperable lung malignancy. The patient has a good history and clinical signs, and so will be a particularly effective case with which to teach your students. He has agreed to help with the session. However, as you approach the bed with your students, he appears to be crying.

Rank in order the following actions in response to this situation
(1 = Most appropriate; 5 = Least appropriate)

A Do not enter the room as he is unlikely to agree to the teaching.

B Explain that emotional turbulence is a normal part of terminal disease.

C Continue as planned to take his mind off his condition.

D Talk to the patient about how he is feeling and whether there is anything you can do to help.

E Ask the patient whether he would be interested in helping you teach medical students.

33. The nurse on the ward wants you to speak to Meredith who has become increasingly anxious about a bilateral mastectomy planned for the following day.

Choose the THREE most appropriate actions to take in this situation

A Encourage Meredith to express her concerns.

B Ask the nurse to identify any problems and get back to you if they are surgical.

C Refer to the psychologist.

D Speak to the family to identify any of the patient's concerns.

E Talk Meredith through the procedure and what will happen afterwards.

F Inform your registrar early on if she appears to show doubt about the procedure.

G Inform Meredith that other patients will have missed out on the operating slot if she changes her mind.

H Tell Meredith she shouldn't worry as breast reconstructions are very good these days.

34. Stephen has recently been diagnosed with congestive heart failure. During a ward round he asks the consultant to explain what this means and the consultant says that you will come back later on for this purpose.

Rank in order the following actions in response to this situation
(1 = Most appropriate; 5 = Least appropriate)

A Tell Stephen that 'heart failure is an inability of the central pump to adequately perfuse the peripheral tissues'.

B Ask what Stephen understands so far and what he wants to know.

C Tell Stephen that 'congestive heart failure' essentially means that the heart isn't working properly.

D Print out a patient information leaflet provided by the Trust.

E Tell Stephen that there are some good websites online and that he should read around the subject once he is discharged.

35. Rachel is being treated for severe renal failure but refuses to accept that she will need dialysis and/or a transplant in future. She says that she would prefer not to know about the disease. Your consultant informs her that it is serious and asks you to reiterate the treatment options and poor prognosis. When you return to speak to Rachel, she appears very happy.

Choose the THREE most appropriate actions to take in this situation

A Inform Rachel that it can be helpful to know what to expect, and to plan treatment, if you are able to discuss the disease with her.

B Encourage her to share how she is feeling about her disease at the moment.

C Inform her family instead about the things that Rachel does not want to know about.

D Place detailed written information on the condition at Rachel's bedside.

E Ask her why she feels happy as it is clearly not appropriate at this time.

F Agree not to discuss the topic any further if she insists on not being told.

G Ask the transplant nurse to approach the topic of prognosis and survival rates.

H Ask one of the nurses who gets on particularly well with Rachel to raise the issue.

36. The palliative care nurse asks you to join her for a meeting with Jenny, whose husband is close to the end of life. You have been on leave for the last two weeks and are not familiar with the patient. Your seniors are all in clinic and you are alone on the ward.

Rank in order the following actions in response to this situation
(1 = Most appropriate; 5 = Least appropriate)

A Agree to see Jenny with the nurse, after reading through the medical notes.

B Ask the nurse to familiarize you with the case details before meeting Jenny.

C Agree to be present during any discussion but not to answer any medical questions.

D Ask the palliative care nurse if she can wait until your seniors are back from clinic as they know the patient better.

E Go into the meeting and pick up the story as the nurse talks to Jenny.

37. The registrar asks you to a book a foot X-ray for a patient on the orthopaedic ward. When booking the scan, you are only able to find an option for 'CT foot'. He asks you to book a CT but call radiology to amend the request. You are apprehensive about this strategy as you have previously seen it lead to inappropriate imaging.

Rank in order the following actions in response to this situation
(1 = Most appropriate; 5 = Least appropriate)

A Book a CT foot and then call radiology to amend your request.

B Voice your concerns and explain that you have seen this strategy fail before.

C Speak with radiology first, and then book the 'CT foot'.

D Complete a clinical incident form about the registrar's willingness to compromise patient safety.

E Ask the registrar to book the scan under his name.

38. Your consultant is about to close the abdomen after a very long emergency laparotomy. He is a formidable personality and earlier told you to stop talking so that he could concentrate on finishing the operation. Although you have not been paying full attention, you think that a swab might have been left behind but are far from certain.

Rank in order the following actions in response to this situation
(1 = Most appropriate; 5 = Least appropriate)

A Immediately inform the consultant of your suspicion.

B Ask the scrub nurse to re-count the swabs.

C Ask another question to 'break the ice', before raising the possibility of a swab being left in the abdomen.

D Remain quiet as you were not really paying attention.

E Ask an indirect question such as: 'How harmful would it be if a swab was left in the abdominal cavity?'

39. Your consultant has agreed to complete a work-based assessment for you on numerous occasions but has not yet done so. The deadline for completion of all assessments is approaching.

Rank in order the following actions in response to this situation
(1 = Most appropriate; 5 = Least appropriate)

A Ask for your consultant's login details to complete the form yourself.

B Find another consultant to complete a work-based assessment.

C Let the foundation school know that you are having difficulty finding assessors.

D Remind your consultant that the deadline is approaching.

E Let your Educational Supervisor know you are having difficulty finding assessors.

40.

You have clerked Mr Smith, a 56-year-old man with abdominal pain, who was also reviewed by Dr Mayer, the duty consultant. The following day, the new duty consultant reads your clerking and proposes a completely different management plan. He has no new information to hand and did not examine the patient, and you are unhappy with his suggestions.

Rank in order the following actions in response to this situation
(1 = Most appropriate; 5 = Least appropriate)

A Politely decline to follow the second consultant's management plan until he sees the patient.

B Clarify with the second consultant to whom you are ultimately responsible.

C Highlight the differences in management between the two consultants.

D Accept the plan instigated by the second consultant.

E Ask the registrar to see the patient afterwards for a 'tie-breaker' opinion.

ANSWERS

1. **B, E, D, C, A**

You must obtain the patient's permission before discussing any confidential information with relatives (B). Once consent has been obtained, it is preferable to share information with the patient and family simultaneously (E). This avoids repetition and minimizes the risk of misunderstandings and/or misinformation. While questions are better answered by the day team, patients and relatives should not be excluded from information over an entire weekend (D). You should not seek to delegate tasks inappropriately to nursing colleagues (C). While it seems compassionate to address the relatives' concerns (A), the patient is your primary concern and therefore his consent is necessary first.

2. **D, A, E, C, B**

Thorough documentation of consent is mandatory (D). Establishing what the patient already knows may allow you to avoid repetition and clarify any misunderstandings (A). It is not usually necessary to insist on a witness being present (E), although this might be worth documenting if one happens to be there. You might wish to speak with a senior (C) before obtaining consent but should be able to manage if you understand and are competent performing the procedure. Legal advice would only be necessary in extreme situations and would usually be sought by a more senior doctor (B).

3. **A, D, C, E, B**

The history is an essential part of any clinical assessment and, if the patient is stable, every effort should be made to obtain one where possible (A). However, this should be balanced against the time available and needs of other patients who might be awaiting your attention (D). It may be necessary to postpone the history until a translator can be found (C) or until a more convenient time (B), although this risks discriminatory treatment. Collateral history from a reliable source (E) may be useful but is not an alternative to completing your own assessment.

4. **B, C, A, D, E**

The success of this interview relies on two factors: whether the patient is happy for her brother-in-law to translate and whether he can do so effectively. You should try to establish, explicitly or through body language, whether she is comfortable with her brother-in-law interpreting (B). It may be possible to re-book the appointment with a translator, but this delays dealing with her medical problem (C). If relying on the brother-in-law, you should reiterate the need for him to translate everything (A). The receptionist may prove to be an ineffective interpreter, further complicate the consultation, and might not be acceptable to the patient (D).

It would be futile to attempt a consultation in the clinic when you are unable to communicate verbally (E).

5. B, F, H

Although alcohol intake my be pertinent to this elective admission, it can be addressed more effectively after the ward round (B). After your initial assessment, it may be advisable to inform your senior (F) and involve an alcohol services representative (H) if the patient agrees. You should not stop a busy ward round to address non-urgent issues (A) (D), blindly prescribe medication for alcohol withdrawal (C), or give the patient instructions without a full history (E). It would be unprofessional and unhelpful to discourage the nurse from sharing important information (G).

6. A, D, E, C, B

You should book the urgent scan immediately (A) and be open about your own error. If the registrar has requested the scan, he should either ensure that you are clear about the reasons or make the request himself (D), or another senior doctor might be able to help (E). Sharing your doubts might be honest but puts the radiologist in the difficult position of receiving conflicting assessments from the clinical team (C). You should accept blame for your own errors and not dishonestly attribute this to colleagues (B).

7. C, D, B, E, A

It is important that doctors do not routinely work beyond their required hours. However, patient safety is paramount and you should be satisfied that the patient is stable before handing tasks over to the on-call doctor (C). It would be helpful to initiate any tasks (e.g. by directing the nursing staff) which can be done before the on-call doctor arrives (D). Staying for 15 minutes might be helpful but only if all urgent tasks can be completed in this time (B). Prioritizing tasks is likely to be outside the nurse's experience and therefore asking her to do this would be an unfair request (E). Leaving the ward without considering the new patient (A) is potentially dangerous and the least appropriate option.

8. A, B, F

An apology may help to appease the situation (A) and the opportunity could be used as learning exercise to obtain feedback on your performance (B). However, you should not be coerced into continuing working in this situation (F), and your only responsibility is to ensure that a thorough and safe handover is completed (E) so that the FY2 can finish the remaining tasks herself (C) (D). It should not be necessary to involve the surgical registrar (G) or consultant (H) unless the situation could not otherwise be resolved.

9. D, A, B, C, E

Use an appropriate model for communicating information over the telephone in the correct order, e.g. SBAR. This stands for Situation—introduction (D) and brief problem; Background—admission diagnosis (A) and relevant past history; Assessment—vital signs, current problem, and management (B); Recommendations—your request (C). There would be no need to call the consultant at home as the registrar has not had a chance to review the case (E).

10. B, D, F

As part of your review, you should include the trend in blood results (D) rather than values from a single day (E), which are less informative. You should also document your current management plan (F). As a junior member of the team, you should avoid commenting on the perceived deficits of colleagues (A) unless limiting yourself to factual statements (B). It is not possible to assess a patient retrospectively (C), and notes should only be written retrospectively if this is made very clear. It is never appropriate to avoid documenting your findings (G) and rarely appropriate to undermine colleagues when talking to patients in this way (H).

11. B, E, H

Play therapists are a particularly effective resource as they can invest appropriate time working with children to facilitate successful procedures (B). Before implementing any intervention, it is necessary to explore any concerns of the parents and/or patient and gain their cooperation (E). It is imperative to establish what the patient can comprehend, as learning difficulties span a vast range of cognitive abilities (H). Tricking the patient into the procedure (A) or attempting it in the middle of the night (C) could jeopardize the relationship between clinicans and patient. It would be sensible to attempt options (B), (E), and (H) before resorting to restraints (D) or sedation (F). Inserting a cannula in parents is unnecessary, and is unlikely to alleviate the child's concerns (G).

12. B, A, E, C, D

A clinician of appropriate experience must consent the patient as usual for her OGD. However, you might be an appropriate person to consent the patient for the additional biopsy and participation in the trial. It is essential that additional consent is obtained, irrespective of her perceived anxieties (B). Consent must be obtained in partnership with patients and you should avoid making assumptions about the information that they want or need (A).

Patients also have a right to refuse or agree to participate in research, and this decision should not be made on their behalf (E). It should be made clear to potential participants that a research intervention is not designed specifically for their benefit but is part of a research programme to benefit similar patients in future (C). Obtaining an additional biopsy without obtaining consent might amount to battery, even if the samples were not used (D).

13. C, B, A, E, D

Ensuring the prompt and effective discharge of patients is an important part of being an FY1. However, the urgent care needs of your patients must be prioritized (C). Colleagues might be able to help, but you should minimize disruption to others by completing the tasks yourself when possible (B). Asking the nurse to contact your senior risks interrupting the medical registrar with a task which you should really complete (A). Although taking two minutes to write a brief discharge letter (E) minimizes time away from unwell patients, it may result in a hastily written and inadequate discharge summary. Nursing staff should not generally complete discharge letters, and signing documentation in advance constitutes very poor clinical practice (D).

14. C, A, D, B, E

It is essential to explore the patient's concerns to address specific anxieties that might underlie his complaints (C). It may be appropriate to support the registrar's actions, although this may appear defensive as an initial response (B). Patients may seek comfort from religious or spiritual leaders, but such an offer should only be made after an attempt to understand your patient's values and beliefs (E). It is possible that the registrar failed to consider appropriate treatment options, in which case the situation might be escalated to a consultant. However, apologizing for the registrar's 'failings' prematurely assigns fault to your senior colleague which may well be unfounded (A). It is not the responsibility of the FY1 to independently refer patients for specialist treatment (D).

15. B, E, A, D, C

It is important to identify whether Tim is aware of the problem and any difficulties which might be impacting on his performance (B). At some point it may be necessary to involve your consultant (E); however, as a fellow FY1 it might be unwise to accuse Tim directly of 'failings' (D). Sharing the additional workload with the other FY1 is not a long-term solution and does not address your late departure from the ward or the difficulties which Tim might be facing (A). It would be inappropriate to act in concert with the other surgical FY1 against Tim, particularly to the detriment of patients (C).

16. C, A, D, B, E

In any scenario where a colleague voices concerns, you should explore these further to identify ways of alleviating the problem (C). The vignette raises the important ethical responsibility that health practitioners have to patients—provided that there is minimal risk to one's own health there is a responsibility to treat all patients equitably (A). If the nurse continued to refuse performing the procedure, you may complete the task yourself (D). It would be unprofessional to demand that the nurse takes the sample or threaten to report her (B) and unfair to ask another nurse to take blood without informing them of the risks (E).

17. B, A, D, C, E

Ward duties must be completed to ensure that patients are safe. In this scenario, you should complete your ward round but postpone any non-urgent discussions until the following day (B). It would be impolite to ignore the family and consent is required before examining patients (A). Unless there was an urgent issue affecting the patient's health, you should delay discussions which might cause you to miss your flight (D). Removing the families (C) is likely to take more time than talking to them and distracts a nurse from their own duties. It would be inappropriate to omit patients from your ward round (E) without at least asking a colleague to review them.

18. **E, C, D, A, B**

GMC guidelines require consent for operations to be taken by someone competent to perform the procedure or an appropriate delegatee. The latter must be sufficiently well informed to act as such, and this is likely to exclude FY1 doctors. In this setting, the task should be deferred to a senior surgeon (E), even at the risk of losing a valuable teaching opportunity. If the registrar is unavailable, you should refuse the request (C) rather than attempting to consent the patient independently (D) (A). Involving the anaesthetist in the consent process for a surgical procedure (B) is inappropriate and unlikely to earn you many friends in theatre!

19. **B, A, D, C, E**

It is important to establish the reasons for the patient's behaviour, irrespective of his previous medical history (B). You should have an open discussion as to the dangers of discharge given his medical history (A). The nursing staff may be inadvertently antagonizing the patient and this should be considered during your assessment (D). Occasionally it can be helpful to involve the next of kin to improve compliance, although this may be difficult without further information or patient consent (C). Finally, you should assist your colleagues and help to ensure the patient's safety regardless of his medical history (E).

20. **A, B, C**

Death certificates must be completed accurately as they are a legal record. Senior members of your team (A) (B) are most likely to have a clear idea of the precise cause. A pathologist (C) could help separate multiple complicated circumstances into causes acceptable to the registrar of deaths. The other people listed might contribute under specific circumstances but would not routinely be contacted to establish cause of death (D) (E) (F) (G) (H).

21. **B, C, E, D, A**

The minimum you should document in the notes is your findings on examination (B). Any clerking requires an objective clinical assessment, and if concerns of neglect were to be raised later on, this would also prove useful. A brief summary of your clinical assessment (C) would help people reading your notes in future but should not replace a full clerking. Documentation must take place and should ideally be contemporaneous to ensure maximum accuracy. You should not usually see other routine cases before writing in the notes for this child (E). Similarly, your assessment does not require input from a senior (D) and in any event should not be modified by anyone else's opinion. Your assessment might be wrong, but should be documented nevertheless. However, you should confine yourself to objective statements and not infer too many details from the parents' appearance (A).

22. **C, B, D, A, E**

Documentation is important but must be prioritized after emergencies. You should attend the crash call, even though other doctors will do so, unless another emergency prevents you from doing so (E) (A).

Although a pyrexial patient alone might not divert you from documenting in the notes, you should see this patient after the crash call (C). This is because by this time there is a risk that they might be deteriorating. You should then return and write in the notes for the patient who fell (B), making clear when you do so that it is a retrospective entry. Although other tasks might arise while seeing the two unwell patients, documentation should be as contemporaneous as possible and every effort must be made to return soon afterwards (D).

23. **B, D, F**

You must review the potentially unwell patient as a priority. Doing so with the medical student will provide an extra pair of hands and a valuable learning opportunity (B) (A). Responsibility for reviewing the patient should not be delegated to the student, even if you soon join him (C). You might then ask the student to place the cannula which should be within his range of experience (D). Although you could site the cannula, this would deprive the student of practice and prevent you from attending to the waiting family (E). You should speak with the patient's family, ideally with a nurse present (F) (G). Although you could speak with the family alone, it is often helpful to have a nursing colleague handy for additional perspective. The family are anticipating a conversation with the medical team and are unlikely to be unimpressed by a medical student (H).

24. **A, F, G**

Effective management of trauma requires a rapid multi-disciplinary approach. This is achieved in most hospitals by putting out a trauma call through the switchboard (F). The trauma team will include a general surgeon, an orthopaedic surgeon, an anaesthetist, and emergency physicians. It will also alert ancillary staff (e.g. the on-call radiographer). There should be no additional need to contact the orthopaedic consultant (B). The facts do not suggest major haemorrhage or haematological complications and so there is not yet a reason to contact the duty haematologist (C).

The trauma team will not routinely include an obstetrician or a neonatologist. Your registrar is contacting obstetrics and so you should contact the neonatology registrar (A). You might also consider sourcing specialist equipment (G) in case an emergency Caesarean section becomes necessary in resuscitation.

The cardiac arrest team will be differently composed to the trauma team (D) and there is no obvious benefit from sourcing a phototherapy light (E). Medical students might like to observe if they are present, but given the circumstances should not be prioritized (H).

25. **B, C, D, E, A**

Other colleagues in the hospital will depend on your answering your bleep promptly. However, this must be balanced against the need to complete tasks which you have already started.

In this case, it would be unfair to subject the patient to a further needle attempt so you can answer the call (A). Therefore you should secure the cannula before answering (B). Alternatively, you could ask someone else to answer the bleep if they are available (C). Although securing the cannula is justifiable, it would be preferable to answer the call before cleaning the area (D), except of course for sharps and clinical waste. Ignoring the bleep is unacceptable (E) and only marginally better than subjecting the patient to further unnecessary needles.

26. **B, D, E, C, A**

Additional steps should be taken to protect any patient who is particularly anxious about confidentiality. A first step might be removing sensitive details from your patient list (B). You should also let other colleagues know that the information is sensitive so that nothing is said inadvertently in front of family members (D). Beyond this, you should respect his confidentiality in the same way as any other patient (E).

You should be able to guarantee confidentiality, and although you can explore reasons for the patient wanting to keep his diagnosis secret, he should not be coerced into telling his family (C). You cannot remove details of an important diagnosis from the patient's medical notes (A) as this information might be necessary to ensure that he is managed appropriately in future.

27. **A, B, C, E, D**

You have a duty to confront behaviour which threatens patient dignity. As Karen is currently speaking to the child in a way that you think is inappropriate, you should raise the issue immediately (A). Alternatively, you might wish to approach the nursing hierarchy instead of speaking to Karen directly (B). However, this would be a more appropriate first step if the behaviour causing you concern had already happened. You should not attempt to investigate Karen's behaviour by talking to other staff (C), which might be seen as gossip or bullying. Informing officials in the Trust might be necessary (E) depending on what was said. However, from the scenario description it would seem fair to escalate concerns within the ward hierarchy before doing so anywhere else. Once you have developed a concern, it should always be acted upon in a way which satisfies you that the issue will not arise again (D).

28. C, B, D, A, E

Your first step should be to gather information in case immediate improvements are possible (C). You might discover that the patient is more interested in communicating her concerns than making a formal complaint per se. However, you might direct her to PALS who can provide further information as well as liaising with the clinical team, especially once she has been discharged (B). Any concerns should be passed on to your consultant again so that improvements can be instigated and a formal complaint anticipated (D).

You should certainly not dissuade the patient from complaining if she believes that she has good reason (A). Suggesting it will make no difference and will also risk undermining the clinical governance process at your Trust. However, equally, you should not incite complaints to generate change that you believe is necessary—your own concerns should be raised openly with the senior team (E).

29. A, B, F

Patient safety is always your priority and this patient should be saved an unnecessary catheterization (A) (D).

Although you are the responsible clinician in this case, you cannot accept full responsibility for the error (G). The student is not yet a doctor, but he must take some responsibility for any procedures he performs. He should have checked the patient's identity and indication before proceeding. For this reason, both you and the student should apologize to the misidentified patient (F). However, it would be unfair to blame the student entirely and mistakes are best learned from by helping to rectify the consequences, not by being sent home (C).

A clinical incident form should then be completed (B) to create a paper trail and in case lessons can be learned for future. You should identify any contributing factors, e.g. a patient in the wrong bed or not wearing a wristband. You should certainly not mislead the patient (E) and there is no clinical indication for an ultrasound KUB (H).

30. A, E, B, C, D

The patient requiring scrotal exploration needs to be consented promptly so that he can be taken to theatre. However, GMC guidance clearly states that the person taking consent should usually be able to perform the procedure themselves. In this case, your registrar is clearly the most appropriate person to take consent once they are available (A). Alternatively, an experienced SHO might be sufficiently experienced to take consent (E). The consultant would clearly have enough experience to consent the patient but contacting him at home is unlikely to persuade him to come in for this purpose (B). The medical registrar is unlikely to offer advice beyond telling you not to take the consent yourself (C). If you were to consent the patient, you could potentially be found to have done so negligently if an issue were to arise afterwards (D).

31. B, C, E

Although the man's tape recorder and aggressive tone apply pressure, you should remain resilient and adhere to the general principles of professionalism.

You should try to ignore the tape recorder (B) and explain that you cannot discuss a patient's care without their consent (C) (F). If he persists and/or is threatening, you might like to ask him to leave and contact security if necessary (E).

Saying 'no comment' is unhelpful (A), as is passing the problem on to a colleague (D) who is unlikely to appreciate the gesture. You should certainly not lie to the relative (G), despite his aggressive tone, or exacerbate the situation by attempting to turn off the tape recorder (H).

32. D, E, B, A, C

Although you are with medical students, this should not stop you exercising compassion when one of your patients is visibly upset. You should leave the students at a distance and ascertain what has happened to lower his mood (D). You may then ask whether this means that he would prefer to delay the teaching session until another day (E). This is preferable to assuming that he will not want to continue (A). Whether or not he wants to continue, you can certainly use this to raise the issue of managing low mood in patients with terminal disease (B). The worst option here would be to ignore his crying and continue the teaching session (C) as this is likely to be awkward for your students and potentially further upsetting for the patient.

33. A, E, F

You should listen to Meredith and try to understand her perspective (A) before talking her through the procedure again with reference to any specific concerns she might have expressed (E). If there is a possibility that she might opt to cancel the procedure, you should speak with your registrar early (F). She might benefit from counselling by a more senior doctor, and cancellations are best anticipated early in case other patients can fill the operating slot. However, you should not coerce the patient's decision (G) or make light of the operation that she is worried about (H). Patient concerns about an operation fall squarely within your remit, and the nursing staff should not be discouraged from contacting you about similar problems in future (B).Speaking to the patient's family (D) or referring her to a psychologist (C) would be presumptuous as you do not know whether this is what she would want.

34. B, D, A, C, E

Ideally, any explanation should start by finding out what your audience already knows (B). This prevents repetition of knowledge and allows you to clarify any specific misunderstandings. Patient information leaflets are helpful (D) because they can be read in the patient's own time and provide clear and accurate information. They are best used as an adjunct to verbal explanation so that patients have an opportunity to ask questions. Although heart failure is inability of the pump to perfuse the tissues, this textbook definition might be lost on a patient hearing it for the first time (A). However, over-simplications can sound frightening (C), and you should beware of letting patients who present with occasional ankle swelling go home thinking that you have diagnosed a terminal illness. Although Stephen should read about heart failure if he wishes, patients can easily become lost in the masses of information available online. Therefore this should not be recommended as a first source of information (E).

35. **A, B, F**

It is important to share information with patients, but only if this is what they want. We should not force information on them anymore than we should force anything else. However, you do have a duty to make sure that Rachel understands why it would be helpful to her to talk about her disease (A). You should try to understand her perspective by listening carefully (B). If she continues to choose not to know, the issue should not be raised again unless there is reason to think that she has changed her mind (F).

You should certainly not coerce her to accept information by providing written leaflets (D) or asking other team members to approach the subject (G) (H). If Rachel consents, you could talk to her family, but in the absence of such an agreement they should not be told anything more than normal (C). It would be callous to obstruct Rachel's happiness by telling her that she should be otherwise (E).

36. **D, A, B, E, C**

Your seniors are better placed to attend this meeting (D) as they will know the patient and might already have a rapport with Jenny. They will also have greater experience with conversations of this nature. If you do attend the meeting, you should certainly familiarize yourself with the patient's notes beforehand (A). Asking the nurse to brief you would be inadequate preparation for such an important meeting (B), as would identifying the issues as the conversation unfolds (E). It would be unhelpful and awkward for all parties if you attended the meeting but declined to contribute (C).

37. **B, C, E, A, D**

You should learn from previous mistakes, whether your own or a colleague's. You will want to let your registrar know that errors have occurred in this way previously (B). He might then amend his strategy or decide that the investigation is sufficiently urgent to proceed with the original plan. Alternatively, you first could check with radiology that this is an appropriate way to order the investigation (C). You should be very cautious if you are doing something that you know might lead to an error (A), and it might be preferable if the registrar formally takes responsibility for requesting the investigation in this way (E). Although it would not be a measured response to complete a clinical incident form, the unclear computer system could benefit from being updated (D).

38. **A, B, C, E, D**

In this unenviable position, you are nevertheless duty bound to raise your concern and should do so with the operating surgeon (A). The scrub nurse should certainly re-count the swabs, but this instruction might be better coming from the surgeon himself (B).

Many studies of human error have found that juniors are too indirect when questioning more experienced colleagues. If you believe that a swab might have been left in the abdomen, you should say so. Asking other questions first (C) or skirting around the issue (E) is likely to try your consultant's patience when a direct question would have been sufficient. The worst option would be to remain quiet, as you might have been the only person with the opportunity to stop the patient undergoing a second operation to remove an aberrant swab (D).

39. **D, B, E, C, A**

Finding people who are sufficiently senior to complete work-based assessments can be difficult. However, these are useful learning experiences and a minimum number are necessary to pass FY1. The Foundation Programme is 'trainee led' which means that you are responsible for finding sufficient learning opportunities and assessors to complete the minimum number. For this reason, you should remind the consultant who promised you a work-based assessment (D). If this is becoming fruitless, you should approach someone else (B). Only in the rare event of you finding yourself in difficulty (i.e. no one willing to complete assessments) should you raise the issue with your Educational Supervisor (E). The foundation school is unlikely to be interested at that time, but might need to consider modifying your post in future if insufficient educational opportunities are available (C). Of course, it would be dishonest to masquerade as your consultant and complete the assessment yourself (A).

40. **C, D, E, B, A**

Management plans change with time according to new information, evolving clinical signs, and the approach of the clinicians involved. It is important that doctors—and particularly consultants—have discretion in managing patients.

However, you should point out the discrepancy between the two plans (C) as this might make the second consultant consider why they differ. If he insists, you should generally implement his plan as he is now ultimately responsible for the patient (D). You should not generally seek an uninvited third opinion with a view to undermining a consultant (E). If you have serious concerns about a new management plan, you should of course raise these and take necessary action to avoid harm occurring. If you are uncertain, your registrar might be able to explain the reason for this new approach. Clarifying to whom you are ultimately responsible might be interpreted as impertinent (B)—you are clinically accountable to the consultant on duty that day.

Although it would be sensible to ask the consultant to see Mr Smith, you should not coerce him to do so by refusing to implement his plan otherwise (A). It is pragmatic to accept that senior doctors will not always review patients before instigating a management plan.

Patient focus

Introduction

Questions within this section assess your ability to keep the patient as the focus of care at all times. To achieve this, you should listen carefully to patients' ideas, concerns, and expectations, and understand that their needs often go beyond a 'positive clinical outcome'. You should always show compassion and respect while working with patients to develop a management plan that suits their needs.

- Patient safety is your first priority, always.
- Patient safety is only part of your responsibility. You should also look out for patients' dignity, convenience, and general well-being.
- Work with patients when developing a treatment plan. Understand their perspective, and then communicate yours clearly.
- Doctors and other healthcare professionals can contribute to the well-being of patients beyond simply treating disease. Good health is a consequence of biomedical, psychological, and social factors.

QUESTIONS

1. Mavis has recently been widowed and has a history of mild dementia. She was admitted several weeks ago with pneumonia, which has gradually resolved. She worked hard with the physiotherapy team and has returned to her functional baseline level of activity. Despite this, her family highlights several concerns which the nurses are keen for you to address before Mavis is discharged.

Rank in order the following actions in response to this situation
(1 = Most appropriate; 5 = Least appropriate)

A Assist Mavis's daughter-in-law, who feels that Mavis requires a lot of help with looking after her bungalow.

B Address her son's concerns about possible financial exploitation by a neighbour.

C Address her brother's concerns that her memory loss is becoming much worse, and she needs further medical treatment.

D Discuss the family's concerns with Mavis, and obtain her perspective first.

E Assist Mavis's nephew who wants her to enter a residential home where she can be supervised, in case she falls.

2. You have arranged some bedside teaching for a group of six medical students with a patient on your ward who is suffering from multiple sclerosis. On arrival you find her to be in emotional distress due to worsening of symptoms and a recent financial dispute with her family. You had previously agreed to spend 45 minutes with the patient and students, and do not have any other patient with whom you could teach the students.

Rank in order the following actions in response to this situation
(1 = Most appropriate; 5 = Least appropriate)

A Teach the students clinical theory in a classroom instead.

B Explain that emotional turbulence is a normal part of chronic disease, and continue with the bedside teaching as planned.

C Attempt teaching, but agree that if she continues to be upset you are happy to discontinue.

D Teach the students a lesson in communication skills by exploring her family issues.

E Ignore the issue altogether and restrict your teaching to brief examination of the patient's neurological system.

3. You are a foundation doctor working in a GP surgery and have spent the morning assessing an infant with possible meningitis, admitting a young man with suicidal ideation, and breaking the news of a pancreatic malignancy to a previously healthy 55-year-old. Prior to your lunchtime home visits, a 60-year-old man visits your practice for the fourth time in two months with generalized worsening 'aches', despite normal examination, investigations, and maximal medical therapy. Your ten-minute consultation fails to assuage him.

Rank in order the following actions in response to this situation (1 = Most appropriate; 5 = Least appropriate)

A Explain that you must see other patients with serious life-threatening conditions, and you do not have the time he requires.

B Ask whether he would be interested in the services of complementary health providers.

C Refer the patient to a rheumatologist.

D Spend 10 minutes focusing on the patient's psychological and social well-being.

E Offer the patient the advice of another doctor at the practice.

4. A patient appears to be worried during your surgical ward round, and the consultant suggests the need to 'get to the bottom of these worries before we explore the different treatment options'. You consider how you might go about doing this.

Rank in order the following actions in response to this situation (1 = Most appropriate; 5 = Least appropriate)

A Allow the patient to express their concerns when they chose and without directly asking.

B Ask the nurse looking after the patient today to explore any concerns.

C Ask the healthcare assistant looking after the patient today to explore any concerns.

D Speak to the family to identify any concerns that the patient may have.

E Set aside 20 minutes to speak with the patient to establish any underlying concerns.

5. One of your patients appears to be very depressed, which she believes to have been precipitated by a recent bereavement. You realize that her loss parallels one of your own experiences and wonder how this might be used to develop rapport with your patient.

Rank in order the following actions in response to this situation
(1 = Most appropriate; 5 = Least appropriate)

A Describe your own loss and subsequent feelings in detail.

B Explain how you can empathize with her because of your own similar loss.

C Acknowledge her understandable sadness from experiencing a personal loss.

D Change the subject, as dwelling on it may make her more upset.

E Encourage her to discuss her feelings with a religious or spiritual leader instead.

6. You are working as an FY1 doctor on the gastroenterology ward. Maureen has early dementia and declines further treatment, despite the medical team's recommendations and her daughter's insistence. Her daughter explains about a previous protracted debate between other doctors and her mother, which led to Maureen eventually being 'overruled', and asks you to avoid a similar delay and initiate treatment straight away.

Rank in order the following actions in response to this situation
(1 = Most appropriate; 5 = Least appropriate)

A Assess Maureen's capacity for refusing this treatment.

B Read through the notes and establish whether Maureen lacks capacity.

C Ask the daughter to help in your assessment of Maureen's capacity.

D Just get on and treat Maureen irrespective of her wishes.

E Avoid the decision and seek the input of a superior.

7. You are seeing Derek, a 45-year-old man. He specifically mentions to you his relative who has recently been diagnosed with cancer. This news has concerned him, and Derek is worried about his own risk of developing cancer. Having done some reading on the internet, he is requesting a full-body CT scan.

Rank in order the following actions in response to this situation
(1 = Most appropriate; 5 = Least appropriate)

A Explain the dangers of X-radiation and the associated increased risk of cancer.

B Explain that his absolute risk of developing cancer is low.

C Take a history and examination.

D Offer a full-body CT scan.

E Prescribe anxiolytics

8. You are reviewing a man who is troubled about his weight. Despite having tried various dieting and exercise plans, he is now requesting medication for weight loss. His body mass index (BMI) is currently 35, and under local policy guidelines he has not yet reached the BMI required to commence this treatment.

Rank in order the following actions in response to this situation
(1 = Most appropriate; 5 = Least appropriate)

A Write him a prescription as he has exhausted alternative options.

B Explain the high cost of this medication, and encourage him to seek it from wholesale online distributors instead.

C Write to the Primary Care Trust (PCT) asking permission to prescribe the medication.

D Inform the patient that he is not of a high enough weight to benefit sufficiently from the medication.

E Refer the patient to another doctor in the practice.

9. You are asked by one of the nursing staff to see Heather, a patient who is refusing elective angiography following a non-ST elevation myocardial infarction.

Rank in order the following actions in response to this situation
(1 = Most appropriate; 5 = Least appropriate)

A Establish her concerns.

B Establish that she has capacity.

C Discuss her decision with family members if Heather agrees.

D Explore alternative treatment options.

E Explain the benefits of the procedure and insist that she must have it done.

10. You are about to share a list of ward jobs after the consultant ward round with your SHO on the oncology ward. You both have plenty of tasks to keep you busy until the end of your shift. The SHO tells you to delay referring Mrs Wilson to the palliative care team until tomorrow, as she is likely to need infusion pumps and will create other tasks which will take too long.

Rank in order the following actions in response to this situation
(1 = Most appropriate; 5 = Least appropriate)

A Complete the list of jobs that your SHO has assigned to you before referring the patient to the palliative team at the end of the day.

B Delegate the task of referring the patient to a nurse although you know that 'doctor to doctor' referrals are expected.

C Complain to your consultant that the SHO is neglecting Mrs Wilson.

D Explain the importance of adequate analgesia in terminal patients to your SHO and suggest that the jobs be reprioritized.

E Follow your colleague's instructions and make the referral to the palliative care team tomorrow.

11. You are working in a genitourinary medicine clinic. A patient attends because she believes that she may have contracted an infection following a recent sexual encounter outside of her long-term relationship.

Choose the THREE most appropriate actions to take in this situation

A Advise her to begin contact tracing, i.e. informing her regular partner.

B Suggest you will have to inform her long-term partner if she does not.

C HIV testing is mandatory.

D Advise a blood test for syphilis antibody.

E Promote safe sexual practices.

F Discuss the morality of multiple sexual partner.s

G Inform the patient's GP to ensure adequate community follow-up.

H Ask a phlebotomist to draw the blood sample to avoid the risk of a needle-stick injury.

12. You have arrived on a ward to review a medical outlier. You retrieve the patient's notes from the treatment room after several wasted minutes searching for them in the notes trolley. You are exasperated as you risk missing lunch, again, if not en route to the canteen within 10 minutes. The telephone at the nurses' station rings. There is no ward clerk. Although the surgical FY1 and his registrar, a staff nurse, and a physiotherapist are standing at the desk, no one answers after 20 rings.

Choose the THREE most appropriate actions to take in this situation

A Tell the surgical FY1 doctor to answer the phone.

B Tell the staff nurse that you are in a great hurry and that she/he should answer the phone.

C Move away from the nurses' station quickly and let the phone be answered by someone else.

D Ask the staff nurse whether you can answer the phone and let her/him know what is needed.

E Pick up the phone and give the handset straight to the staff nurse saying 'It's for you'.

F Ask people at the desk whether someone is waiting for a call and answer the phone if no one volunteers.

G Ask the nurse in charge whether is a policy on answering phones on the ward.

H State to all around the desk that the call might be very important for a relative/carer or directly related to patient care.

13. During your first month working on the neurosurgery ward, you have become increasingly troubled by your registrar's ability. You have seen him misinterpret basic clinical signs. On one occasion you tried to share your concerns with the consultant in charge but he discounted them, highlighting the registrar's natural ability in the operating room.

Rank in order the following actions in response to this situation
(1 = Most appropriate; 5 = Least appropriate)

A Ask your consultant again to consider the registrar's overall performance.

B Inform your Educational Supervisor.

C Approach the registrar, and ask him whether he would be willing to receive teaching from you after work.

D Inform the Clinical Director.

E Share your thoughts with the FY1 on the ward.

14. You are the paediatric FY1 doctor. A nurse asks if you could speak with the family of a 13-year-old patient, Lenka, who does not speak any English. Lenka's family are very angry, and demand that she is moved away from the neighbouring patient who has been coughing vigorously throughout the night. You also notice that Lenka appears to be upset.

Choose the THREE most appropriate actions to take in this situation

A Acknowledge the family's concern, and try to move the patient into a side room.

B Explain to the patient's family the low risk of contracting an infection from neighbouring patients in open bays on the ward.

C Try to establish Lenka's concerns.

D Try to address the concerns of Lenka's family first.

E Ask the neighbouring patient if they would be willing to move into a side room.

F Provide the patient and her family with face masks.

G Ask the ward nurse to address these nursing concerns.

H Provide the neighbouring patient with a face mask.

15. You are clerking patients in the Medical Admissions Unit (MAU). A former colleague approaches and informs you that his father is one of the patients waiting to be clerked. He asks you to see his father first.

Rank in order the following actions in response to this situation
(1 = Most appropriate; 5 = Least appropriate)

A Report your medical colleague to his Educational Supervisor.

B Refuse your colleague's request outright.

C Ask the registrar whether he has any preference for which patient you should see next, and if not, begin with your colleague's father.

D See your colleague's father last, as punishment for his unfair request.

E Establish if there is any particular reason why he wants you to see his father straight away.

16. Lucy is a 24-year-old with Crohn's disease. On reviewing her drug chart, you find that multiple doses of medication have not been given. On questioning the nurse who has been looking after Lucy since her admission, she says that the patient has been refusing to take the medication when offered. However, you have always found the patient to be pleasant and cooperative. Lucy denies being offered any medication by the nurse.

Rank in order the following actions in response to this situation
(1 = Most appropriate; 5 = Least appropriate)

A Report the nurse to the Royal College of Nursing.

B File a clinical incident form for failing to satisfactorily encourage Lucy to take her medication.

C Suggest that the nurse sits with Lucy and encourages her to take her medication.

D Change all her medication to intravenous forms.

E Inform the Ward Sister that Lucy has not been receiving her medications, and ask her to investigate further.

17. Mr Stevenson has recently been diagnosed with terminal mesothelioma. During his admission for a chest infection, you are handed an indefinite DNACPR (Do Not Attempt Cardio-Pulmonary Resuscitation) order that has been in place since a previous admission. On speaking to Mr Stevenson and his family, they do not appear to be aware that this order is in place.

Rank in order the following actions in response to this situation
(1 = Most appropriate; 5 = Least appropriate)

A Tear up the DNACPR order.

B Explain the futility of cardiopulmonary resuscitation in Mr Stevenson's case as the logic of the DNACPR order.

C Apologize for the insufficient explanation given by Mr Stevenson's previous clinicians.

D Inform your registrar.

E Do not inform Mr Stevenson and his family about the DNACPR order at this time, but wait to discuss the matter with Mr Stevenson alone.

18. You are taking a history from the mother of 11-year-old Clara who has presented with shoulder pain. When you are left alone with Clara, she admits that her mother often gets upset with her, and has occasionally hit her in the past. The mother has appeared completely appropriate in her interaction with Clara.

Rank in order the following actions in response to this situation
(1 = Most appropriate; 5 = Least appropriate)

A Clara is most likely referring to reasonable chastisement, and the issue should not be pursued.

B Confront Clara's mother about the accusation, and ask her to volunteer any explanations.

C Document the comments clearly, and attempt to gain more information from Clara, alone if possible.

D Begin a thorough head-to-toe examination of Clara once her mother has returned and, if asked, explain that you are looking for bruises.

E Inform the police.

19. You are about to discharge Terence following his admission for treatment for recurrent epileptic seizures. On getting up to leave the bedside, you overhear his wife's surprise at the doctors allowing him to return to work as a heavy goods vehicle driver. You are confident that Terence has no intention of relinquishing his driving responsibilities, despite promises to the contrary.

Rank in order the following actions in response to this situation
(1 = Most appropriate; 5 = Least appropriate)

A Seek assurances from Terence's wife that he will not return to work.

B Inform Terence's GP.

C Ask Terence to sign an agreement not to return to work in the medical notes.

D Disclose his diagnosis to the Driving and Vehicle Licensing Agency (DVLA).

E You are not responsible for the patient's actions once you have appropriately instructed him.

20. A 40-year-old mother of two children stops you as you are walking by her side room and asks to speak with you. She is visibly worried about the results of her pancreatic biopsy, and asks 'What will happen if I have cancer?'

*Rank in order the following actions in response to this situation
(1 = Most appropriate; 5 = Least appropriate)*

A Reassure the patient that the medical team will do everything they can to try and treat her.

B Reassure her that everything will be fine.

C Ask the patient to wait and ask your senior any questions.

D Echo her concern: 'I can see that you are worried that you might have cancer.'

E Do not say anything, but instead look away in an effort to communicate the grave nature of her problem non-verbally.

21. Iris is 87 and one of your patients on the care of the elderly ward. She has mild dementia but tells you that she doesn't like being dressed by the nursing staff each morning. At home, her carer just stands by in case she needs help, although she concedes that this 'takes longer' than allowing her to dress herself.

*Rank in order the following actions in response to this situation
(1 = Most appropriate; 5 = Least appropriate)*

A Tell Iris that as soon as she goes home she'll be able to go back to her old routine.

B Tell Iris that she can dress herself each morning if she prefers, with help if necessary.

C Pass on Iris's request to the Ward Sister and ask that it be passed on during the nursing handover.

D Explain that this is probably not possible as the nursing staff are busiest in the mornings.

E Tell Iris that you can't interfere with how the ward is run.

22. You are asked by the nurses to site a urethral catheter for Arthur who is an elderly man who needs to urinate frequently. He has known prostate trouble and reduced mobility. It takes at least 5 minutes to get him to the toilet, after which he often does not need to urinate after all.

Rank in order the following actions in response to this situation
(1 = Most appropriate; 5 = Least appropriate)

A Ask Arthur for his views and whether he is troubled about multiple visits to the toilet.

B Offer other options such as a commode or a convene catheter.

C Speak to the urology team to ask if there is anything further that can be done to minimize Arthur's lower urinary tract symptoms.

D Explain the problem to Arthur and then insert a urethral catheter once he consents.

E Tell Arthur that he needs a urethral catheter and then site it carefully.

23. You arrive on the ward one morning to find a student nurse washing a male patient with the curtains open. The patient does not appear to be obviously concerned.

Rank in order the following actions in response to this situation
(1 = Most appropriate; 5 = Least appropriate)

A Pull the curtains closed.

B Ask the patient for his preference and leave the curtains open if he chooses.

C Explain the need to ensure patient privacy to the student nurse afterwards if she is unclear.

D Tell the student nurse in front of the patient that she should learn to respect privacy.

E Carry on with your job as there is not a problem and you shouldn't interfere.

24. You are on a fast-paced surgical ward round. Your consultant tells a patient that she will need a 'Hartmann's procedure which will leave a colostomy' and she signs a consent form. You can tell from her body language that she wants to ask questions but does not feel able to do so.

Rank in order the following actions in response to this situation
(1 = Most appropriate; 5 = Least appropriate)

A Explain that you will come back after the ward round in case she wants to ask any more questions.

B Insist that the consultant stays until he has answered her questions.

C Tell the patient that your consultant will come back later to answer questions.

D Let the ward round continue but remain behind to draw a picture for the patient illustrating Hartmann's procedure.

E Continue with the ward round but return later to answer questions.

25. As you are sitting at the nurses' station completing a discharge summary, you see a 55-year-old patient walking away from you with his gown flapping open at the back.

Rank in order the following actions in response to this situation
(1 = Most appropriate; 5 = Least appropriate)

A Shout to the patient by name so that he can be alerted to his state of undress.

B Catch up with the patient and let him know that he is partially undressed.

C Help him tie up the gown correctly.

D Find a nurse and let them know the patient needs assistance.

E Catch up with the patient and tell him that he should be more careful in case he embarrasses other patients or visitors.

26. Your Trust occasionally authorizes use of protective mittens for certain patients. These are large gloves which essentially prevent patients from using their hands. You are asked to prescribe mittens for a patient out of hours and agree to do so only under specific conditions.

*Rank in order the following actions in response to this situation
(1 = Most appropriate; 5 = Least appropriate)*

A The patient is confused.

B The patient lacks capacity.

C The patient lacks capacity and is at risk of pulling out essential lines and tubes.

D The patient lacks capacity and has pulled out lines and tubes, and alternative strategies have been unsuccessful.

E The patient lacks capacity and is at risk of pulling out essential lines and tubes. The patient's next of kin are fiercely opposed to the use of mittens.

27. A patient admitted to your ward with pneumonia is shown to have tuberculosis (TB). He is asked to wear a face mask when he leaves his side room and told that the case must be reported to the Health Protection Agency. He refuses to allow information about his illness to be sent externally and is often seen outside his side room without a mask.

*Rank in order the following actions in response to this situation
(1 = Most appropriate; 5 = Least appropriate)*

A Explore the reasons for this patient's non-compliance.

B Explain that TB is potentially dangerous and very easily spread to others in the hospital.

C Explain that you will not send his details externally but that his GP must be informed.

D Explain to the patient but submit his details to the Health Protection Agency regardless of whether he gives consent.

E Discharge the patient from hospital without further treatment as he is a danger to other patients.

28. Ron is an elderly man with bowel obstruction. He is delirious and keeps pulling out intravenous cannulas as well as occasionally tugging on his nasogastric tube. Re-inserting cannulas is becoming increasingly time-consuming and he is running out of suitable veins.

Rank in order the following actions in response to this situation
(1 = Most appropriate; 5 = Least appropriate)

A Re-site cannulas in areas less likely to be disrupted (e.g. feet).

B Prescribe gloves/mittens according to hospital policy.

C Try taping and bandaging tubes for additional security.

D Ask whether a 'special' nurse can be assigned for one-to-one care.

E Tape incontinence pads around Ron's hands to stop him pulling out lines.

29. Ivy has severe dementia and often screams out all night. Her clinical condition has recently improved and she has become mobile by 'furniture walking' around the ward. She is violent and abusive when stopped by members of staff.

Rank in order the following actions in response to this situation
(1 = Most appropriate; 5 = Least appropriate)

A Try to reason with Ivy, explaining as far as possible that it is unsafe for her to move around the ward.

B Suggest distracting interventions, such as playing music.

C Prescribe 'as required' (PRN) sedation.

D Ask whether a 'special' nurse can be assigned for one-to-one care.

E Prescribe sedation when Ivy becomes particularly agitated and endangers herself or others.

30. You are hoping to finish your ward round quickly before meeting your Educational Supervisor an hour later. You see Rose, who is very overweight and disabled with osteoarthritis, sitting in a chair. You are told that she developed severe abdominal pain overnight and so will need to be examined in bed. This will require considerable time as she must be hoisted.

Rank in order the following actions in response to this situation
(1 = Most appropriate; 5 = Least appropriate)

A Ask the nursing staff if they can help Rose into bed while you see other patients first.

B Ask Rose whether she would mind lying in bed so that you can examine her thoroughly.

C See Rose later as you are pressed for time.

D See Rose now but feel her abdomen while she is sitting in the chair instead.

E Miss your meeting as your ward round overruns because of this complication.

31. Flora is 73 and suffering from hospital-acquired pneumonia. She has been receiving intravenous antibiotics, but is no longer confused and is becoming unhappy with your continued attempts at cannulation.

Choose the THREE most appropriate actions to take in this situation

A Tell Flora that she will probably die without intravenous antibiotics.

B Stop the antibiotics and re-site the cannula if Flora deteriorates without them.

C Prescribe oral antibiotics and document clearly that Flora refused cannulation.

D Offer to ask a colleague to try if the next attempt fails.

E Explain carefully why a cannula is necessary.

F Tell Flora that the next attempt will be successful.

G Persist with cannulation attempts as Flora does not have capacity.

H Consider whether antibiotics can be de-escalated to oral equivalents.

32. Randhir is 50 and was admitted under the orthopaedic team with severe back pain. MRI shows only degenerative change. Your consultant says that the patient cannot be kept in hospital 'for ever' because of pain and should be discharged with spine surgeon follow-up. The patient and his family do not believe that he can go home because he cannot work and is in severe pain.

Choose the THREE most appropriate actions to take in this situation

A Delete the patient from your list so that he can stay in hospital for a few more days without your consultant knowing.

B Explore Randhir's concerns about going home.

C Promise that you will ensure that the back pain appointment is made within two weeks.

D Tell Randhir that the bed is needed for more urgent cases.

E Carefully explain the nature of mechanical back pain

F Ensure that the pain team is involved with discharge planning so that appropriate analgesia can be provided in the community.

G Prescribe 'as required' (PRN) oramorph until the patient is discharged.

H Tell Randhir he needs to learn to accept the pain as there may be nothing that can be done to help.

33. Archie is a 70-year-old man admitted six days previously for an acute coronary syndrome. He has always been polite and pleasant to speak to. However, today he seems unwilling to answer questions directly and you find yourself becoming increasingly annoyed about having to repeat every question to keep him on track.

Choose the THREE most appropriate actions to take in this situation

A Calculate an Abbreviated Mental Test Score (AMTS)

B Tell Archie that you will come back later after you have seen some other patients.

C Document in the notes that Archie is a 'difficult patient'.

D Consider requesting blood tests, urinalysis, and a chest X-ray.

E Just 'eyeball' Archie the following day rather than seeing him thoroughly on the ward round as this took a long time the day before.

F Take a full history and examine Archie even if it is taking longer than usual.

G Ask your consultant if Archie can be discharged soon as he seems to be fed up with being in hospital.

H Move on quickly so that you can continue the ward round.

34. The nurses inform you that one of your patients has died. He had metastatic lung cancer and had been 'do not resuscitate' for weeks. As you arrive at the patient's side room to confirm death, you are aware that the patient's family are all present, having been called by the Ward Sister.

Choose the THREE most appropriate actions to take in this situation

A Go straight into the room in case another FY1 gets there first.

B Explain why you have arrived and what you intend to do.

C Ask the relatives to leave as there is a bed crisis and the patient has to be moved to the mortuary.

D Ask everyone present for identification to prove they are close relatives.

E Give the relatives some space and come back later, introducing yourself if they are still there.

F Tell the relatives this is probably what the patient 'would have wanted'.

G Let the relatives choose whether to be in the room or outside while you confirm death.

H Enter the room and commence chest compressions if the patient is pulseless.

35. Mike is an intravenous drug user on the gastroenterology ward with liver failure secondary to hepatitis C. He is currently pre-scribed intravenous methadone, but healthcare staff are struggling to administer this as his veins are over-used. He wants to inject his own methadone as he would do at home.

Choose the THREE most appropriate actions to take in this situation

A Discuss with the Ward Sister as to whether self-injecting is acceptable on the ward.

B Explain that it is never acceptable for patients to administer their own medication.

C Ensure that Mike is familiar with the NHS equipment and safety rules (e.g. sharps disposal).

D Offer Mike Oramorph if he agrees to forgo methadone injections

E Only agree if the procedure is supervised by a member of staff.

F Explain that this is not possible as he is hepatitis C positive.

G Give Mike a supply of needles and tell him to 'make himself at home'.

H Ask Mike what dose of methadone he usually takes and prescribe this amount.

36. Roger was admitted to your ward following a stroke which has left him with severe weakness down his left side. He was referred to a local rehabilitation hospital three weeks ago and is currently waiting for a bed to become available.

Choose the THREE most appropriate actions to take in this situation

A Ask the ward physiotherapists if they could spend extra time with Roger before a rehabilitation bed becomes available.

B Ensure that daily inflammatory markers are sent in case Roger develops hospital-acquired pneumonia.

C Call the rehabilitation hospital and insist that they find a bed as Roger is at risk of complications (e.g. pressure sores).

D Cross off the routine prescription for daily low molecular weight heparin to reduce the number of injections he receives.

E Call the rehabilitation hospital to check Roger's position on the waiting list and ensure that they know that he has waited for three weeks.

F Keep Roger informed of his progress up the waiting list.

G Discharge Roger home to bypass the rehabilitation hospital.

H Suggest that Roger's family keep calling the rehabilitation hospital to push his name further up the waiting list.

37. Tom is a bus driver admitted with an epileptiform seizure. Your consultant tells Tom that he must inform the DVLA. Later in the day, Tom says that he can't tell the DVLA as driving is his job and he has never had a seizure before this one.

Choose the THREE most appropriate actions to take in this situation

A Call his employer anonymously to let them know he is unsafe to drive.

B Tell Tom that you must inform his employer and call them even if he refuses consent.

C Document clearly any driving advice given to Tom.

D Agree that he is probably not a danger but tell Tom that he should probably let the DVLA know anyway.

E Call the DVLA anonymously but keep this from Tom so that your relationship is not disrupted.

F Explain that there is a reasonable possibility of a second seizure.

G Ask Tom's wife to bring in his driving licence and surrender this to the Ward Sister.

H Explain that you will have to contact the DVLA if he refuses.

38. A staff nurse approaches you with concerns about Mark, a young man with a recently repaired femoral fracture. He insists on wearing his own clothes and will not change into a hospital gown. Friends also bring food in for him (e.g. take-away curries), which upsets other patients.

Choose the THREE most appropriate actions to take in this situation

A Ask Mark to change into a gown because otherwise he is difficult to examine.

B Tell the nurse that there is no good reason why Mark shouldn't wear his own clothes.

C Explain to the nurse that Mark should be able to eat food from outside if he prefers.

D Tell Mark that if he is well enough to eat curry then he is well enough to be discharged.

E Tell the nurse that the other patients should ask their friends/relatives to bring in food if that's what they want.

F Ask Mark to consider other patients having to eat hospital food before choosing food for his friends to bring.

G Suggest that Mark be swapped with another patient who is currently in a side room with diarrhoea and vomiting.

H Tell the nurse that sister controls the ward and that she should speak to Mark if there is a problem.

39. You are asked to site a cannula in John, a patient with traumatic brain injury and a permanent GCS of 8. He is dehydrated and requires intravenous fluid.

Choose the THREE most appropriate actions to take in this situation

A Explain to the patient what you are going to do.

B Aim blind if you can't see a target vein as multiple attempts are unlikely to cause pain.

C Ask a medical student to insert the cannula as he can try a few times and it will be good practice.

D Defer the job until later as it is uncomfortable being in the room with someone who is unresponsive.

E Omit washing your hands and cleaning the area as the patient is unlikely to comment.

F Warn the patient about a 'sharp scratch' as you would for any other.

G Explain to the patient why a cannula is necessary.

H Try to give oral fluid instead to see if this is tolerated.

40. You are on your way to the blood gas analyser with a sample which shouldn't be left out for more than 10 minutes. You hear a patient shouting and put your head around the curtain. An elderly patient of the opposite sex you haven't met before says they have been sitting on the commode for half an hour and shouting to be helped into bed.

Choose the THREE most appropriate actions to take in this situation

A Tell the patient you are in a hurry.

B Tell the patient you are in a hurry but will come back in 10 minutes.

C Offer to help if you can without compromising the sample.

D Say you will let a nurse know that they need help.

E Reassure the patient that someone will probably come to their assistance soon.

F Suggest that the patient pulls the emergency bell to attract the nurses' attention.

G Say you are sorry that they have been there for so long.

H Tell the patient that they shouldn't shout unless there is an emergency as they alarmed you.

ANSWERS

1. D, C, B, A, E

Doctors must work in their patients' interests (D), while respectfully considering the valuable input of family and friends. First, it is essential to gain Mavis's perspective on each concern to assess the need for intervention. You could address her brother's concerns by assessing her mental state using a validated scoring method (e.g. Mini Mental State Examination) and asking the GP to follow up this assessment after discharge (C). Genuine concerns of financial exploitation can be addressed through liaison with your local vulnerable adults' nurse (if applicable) or social worker, but would not usually be managed by a foundation doctor (B). An assessment by the occupational therapist usually identifies and addresses any potential problems with ability to function at home (A). There is no objective evidence of falls and, in any event, a residential home would not be the first step (E) to avoiding these in future.

2. A, C, B, E, D

Foundation doctors show respect for their patients at all times. While it is unfortunate to compromise your teaching commitments, in this instance it would be discourteous and improper to insist on using the patient for your bedside teaching if she was particularly upset. Therefore the classroom option (A) would be preferable.

It is clear that she is already upset, but if the teaching were to continue it would be sensible to identify any deterioration in mood and discontinue the session (C).

It may be socially awkward to ignore obvious signs of distress (E), and a brief clinical examination will be of limited use to your students.

While the environment may provide an authentic example for demonstrating effective communication skills, it would be unfair to subject the patient to this treatment unnecessarily (D). Continuing your teaching as planned would be less inappropriate as it would not be as intrusive as exploring her family issues in front of an audience (B).

3. D, E, B, C, A

Your previous clinical encounters during the day are irrelevant to the care you should provide to this patient. Informing your patient about more 'serious' cases would be the least appropriate option (A). In any frequently attending patient, it is important to address their background and beliefs to identify any underlying concerns which might be bringing them back (D). Of course, it is also possible that they would benefit from another practitioner's insight (E). It is possible that the patient may wish to see a complementary health service provider (B), and such an option might be suggested to appropriate patients. In view of the negative examination and investigations, a rheumatologist is unlikely to offer further insight into the patient's problems (C).

4. E, B, C, D, A

It is your responsibility to work in partnership with your patients and establish and maintain effective relationships with them (E). In this scenario, at the direct request of your consultant, it would be inadvisable to wait and see whether the patient volunteers information themselves (A). Deferring the task to a nurse or healthcare assistant becomes increasingly inappropriate with more limited clinical experience (B, C). It may be appropriate to approach family members, but only once a thorough attempt has been made to discuss the concerns with the patient first and probably only with the patient's consent (D).

5. C, B, A, D, E

In caring for any patient, you should show compassion and develop rapport whilst maintaining a professional adequate distance. This balance is most easily struck by acknowledging her personal loss (C). The appropriateness of disclosing information about yourself is context-specific, but should be avoided if the same goal can be achieved without doing so (B). Explaining your own experiences may jeopardize your professional relationship and shifts the focus away from the patient's problems (A). Acknowledging this event is more likely to be helpful than detrimental, even if she is initially upset (D). Your role as a doctor in this case is to assess her mental state, and a spiritual leader is unlikely to achieve this result. Although such services should be available if requested, you should avoid presuming to understand any patient's specific values or beliefs (E).

6. A, E, B, C, D

The patient's wishes must always be followed, even when contrary to their perceived best interests, provided that the patient has capacity to make their own decisions. No diagnosis (e.g. dementia) precludes a patient having capacity, which therefore must be assessed (A). It is appropriate to seek the advice of a senior depending on the gravity of the decision being made (E). Because capacity is time- and decision-specific, you cannot rely on previous clinical assessments of Maureen's capacity (B). It would be inappropriate to involve a third party in this decision which should be the responsibility of the medical team (C). Any treatment given contrary to a competent patient's wishes may constitute battery (D).

7. B, C, A, E, D

This question requires you to address patient concerns while also providing reassurance when appropriate. Derek has not offered a suitable indication a CT scan, and this should be avoided for reasons of his safety and equitable resource allocation (D). It would be sensible to begin by reassuring Derek that his risk of cancer is very low (B). You could then reinforce this message by performing a brief systems review and physical examination (C). It is important to explain the risks and benefits of Derek's request, and this includes the dangers of unnecessary exposure to radiation (A). To prescribe Derek anxiolytics as a first-line treatment suggests an inadequate effort to address his underlying concerns (E).

8. **D, C, E, A, B**

GMC guidance states that drugs should be prescribed to meet the needs of patients and not simply because patients demand them (A). It would be even more inappropriate to encourage him to purchase the medication himself from an unlicensed pharmacist (B). GMC guidance requires open and honest practice, discussion of the decision-making process with patients, and prioritization of patients and their treatment (D). Doctors should be familiar with local and national policies that set out agreed criteria for access to particular treatments. The PCT is unlikely to amend its decision in this case (C). Referring the patient to another doctor is unlikely to solve the problem and risks introducing 'false hope' for the patient and wasting another clinician's time (E).

9. **A, B, D, C, E**

It is necessary to foster a professional relationship with every patient by establishing rapport and understanding their particular beliefs (A). It may then be necessary to explore alternatives, first with the patient and then, if appropriate, with family members (D) (C).

Capacity is worth thinking about (B), but should be presumed to be present unless there is reason to believe otherwise (e.g. cognitive impairment). Simply disagreeing with the medical team should not be sufficient to trigger assessment of capacity.

It is never appropriate to insist on a patient having a treatment (E) unless they do not have capacity and a 'best interests' decision has been made. Instead, the pros and cons of each option should be discussed with the patient.

10. **D, A, B, E, C**

Good Medical Practice reminds us to work with colleagues effectively to best serve patient's interests. In this scenario, the SHO has erred in delaying the palliative care referral because of time pressures and you should raise this concern with him first (D). Referring the patient at the end of the day risks them not being seen until the following day and may leave them in pain for longer (A). A nurse may be able to arrange a referral, depending on local policy, but this is otherwise inappropriate (B). Finding your consultant to express concerns is unlikely to lead to a faster palliative care referral for the patient (E) and risks jeopardizing your professional relationship with the SHO (C).

11. **A, D, E**

Confidentiality is central to the trust between patients and doctors. The disclosure of information in the interest of public safety is a complex issue, requiring a balanced and thoughtful clinical judgement in discussion with the patient. In this scenario, it is recommended to complete a sexual diseases screening to rule out common or serious infections (D), although no disease *must* be tested for (C). It would be unfair to defer phlebotomy to another healthcare professional (H) simply because you are worried. At this stage, it is not appropriate to consider disclosure of the patient's sexual encounter to her partner or GP (B) (G), although she might be encouraged to share this information herself (A). Such clinical encounters provide the opportunity to promote safe sexual practices (E), but personal opinions about patients' sexual practices should remain private (F).

12. D, F, H

This common scenario represents many priorities which must be balanced, the most important of which is patient care. The call might be important (H) and should be answered. Ward telephones should be answered promptly even if it is not an individual's direct responsibility because they carry a bleep. The staff nurse may be more persuaded to help if you have their prior agreement (D). It might just be easier to answer the phone quickly, work out what the call is about, and move on (F). You may have unrealistically expected to see a patient within 10 minutes as well as making it to lunch on time. It is often useful to lead by example, in which case simply expecting others to act may be unhelpful (A) (B) (C). Only if the difficulty persists and/or this is a ward that you are likely to visit again should you need to find out the policy on answering telephones (G). Giving the handset directly to the staff nurse (E) would be bad manners and unlikely to provoke a positive response, particularly as you do not know the urgency of the task he is currently managing.

13. A, B, E, D, C

You must ensure patient safety by raising your concerns. In this scenario, it would be most appropriate to approach your consultant again and reiterate your concerns with specific examples of what you believe has been done incorrectly (A). It is possible that your assessment is inaccurate or disproportionate, and discussion with a senior colleague may be helpful in this respect. In any event, if the evidence is unequivocal, the registrar will benefit from the input of a senior clinician rather than a junior colleague (B) (E). It may eventually be appropriate to inform the Clinical Director, although you should escalate stepwise through the local hierarchy (D). Finally, offering clinical teaching to your senior is unlikely to be acceptable to the registrar and would not adequately address any failures on his part to address clinical competencies (C).

14. B, C, D

Good Medical Practice reminds us to listen to patients, and to spend time with relatives and respond to their concerns and preferences. In this scenario, where the child does not speak English, you should try to understand their particular health beliefs before communicating via them with Lenka to identify her concerns (C) (D). The family may be unsettled by conditions on the ward, but the neighbouring patient is unlikely to pose a risk to Lenka (B) and any patients who are at risk of transmitting infectious diseases would already be isolated. Therefore it is unnecessary and an inappropriate use of resources to isolate Lenka or the neighbouring patient, or to provide face masks (A) (E) (F) (H). Since you have begun to speak to the patient's family, and can respond to their concerns, it would be unfair to refer them to the ward nurse (G).

15. **E, C, B, A, D**

The GMC requires doctors to treat patients fairly and not to discriminate unfairly between them. In this instance, your colleague may be abusing his position to gain preferential treatment, but it is possible that his professional insight has raised a concern which *should* expedite his father's care (E). You might benefit from some additional insight from your registrar to help triage the patients waiting to be clerked (C). To refuse your colleague's request outright, without any further questioning, would be ill-mannered (B). To report your colleague at this difficult moment is particularly unfair (A), and to compromise the patient's care would clearly be incorrect (D).

16. **E, C, B, A, D**

Failing to give Lucy her medications could put her at unacceptable risk. There is a clear suggestion that the nurse has neglected an important duty, and the Ward Sister should be requested to investigate the matter further (E). You might try to offer techniques to encourage Lucy to take her medication, but if the nurse has been failing to offer it this is unlikely to address the problem effectively (C). It may become necessary to submit a clinical incident form, but this is unlikely to resolve Lucy's immediate problem (B). Reporting the nurse to an external body would not be your responsibility, and any concerns are reported to the Nursing and Midwifery Council, not the Royal College of Nursing (A). Changing the medication to intravenous forms introduces unnecessary risk to the patient, and does not adequately address the failure by the nurse to give Lucy her medications (D).

17. **D, E, B, C, A**

In this scenario it is essential that there is adequate communication between patient and the clinical team. The revelation that Mr Stevenson and his family do not know about the DNACPR order warrants urgent discussion with your senior (D), and it is not your responsibility to implement any new action or discuss the matter independently (A) (C). It is possible that Mr Stevenson does not want his family to be aware of his agreement not to be resuscitated, and you may gain additional insight through discussion with the patient alone (E). The DNACPR instruction may be appropriate, in which case its reasons and significance warrant explanation (B).

18. **C, B, D, E, A**

Although Clara's description may represent reasonable chastisement, the issue should be pursued as it might indicate non-accidental injury (A). Accurate contemporaneous documentation is key (C) as such cases might be followed up by external agencies and your information relied upon in court. It is not ideal to confront the mother alone (B), particularly at such an early stage. Although a thorough examination is required, informing Clara's mother that you are looking for bruises is likely to antagonize her and would raise the issue inappropriately (D). It may be necessary to inform the police at a later stage, but usually this would only happen after discussion with your seniors (E).

19. D, B, A, C, E

Although confidentiality is necessary to maintain patient trust in doctors, it may be breached to protect others from serious harm. Terence has a legal duty to inform the DVLA, which is likely to ask him to surrender his licence. You may have a professional duty (E) to inform the DVLA if, after discussion with Terence, you believe that he will continue to drive (D).

You could inform Terence's GP who may be able to speak with him further, but they should not be asked to contact the DVLA on your behalf (B). Explaining the issue to Terence's wife may be enough to stop him from driving, but does not provide any guarantee (A). Asking Terence to sign an agreement would be unusual and provides no additional guarantee that he will not continue to work (C).

20. A, C, D, E, B

It is often necessary to strike a careful balance between reassurance and fostering a realistic outlook that does not compromise the patient's faith in the profession. At this stage you cannot fully reassure the patient (B). However, you can guarantee that she will be appropriately looked after regardless of the outcome (A). Deferring her question to a senior (C) is likely to leave her worried and is unnecessary unless you know that the result is 'cancer' and a more senior doctor is required to break bad news. Echoing patient's concerns can be an effective tool for reflective listening and developing rapport but is less appropriate in this example (D). Looking away from the patient would not convey any additional information (E) and might leave her unnecessarily worried.

21. B, C, A, D, E

All healthcare professionals should respect patient autonomy and empower patients as far as possible. Iris should be reassured that she can dress herself if she prefers to do so (B). The request should then be communicated to the nursing staff so that anyone looking after Iris knows her preference (C). Reassuring Iris that her routine will return to normal after leaving hospital is acceptable (A) but should not be used to overlook her preference. The nursing staff might be busy but should not (and are unlikely to) object to helping Iris in this way (D). It would be unhelpful to obviate responsibility for communicating Iris' wishes to the nursing staff (E).

22. A, B, C, D, E

You should only offer invasive treatment if it is in the patient's interest and you have consent. Catheterizing a patient simply for staff convenience would not be appropriate. However, if Arthur is bothered by frequent visits to the toilet, catheterization might become more acceptable (A). Arthur should be made aware of alternatives which are less invasive (B) and other options should be explored for symptom control if possible (C). If catheterization is judged appropriate, and Arthur consents, a catheter may be sited (D). You should not simply tell Arthur he 'needs' a catheter as this is untrue, at least until all other steps have been completed (E).

23. A, C, B, E, D

You should take steps to protect patient dignity whenever possible. In this case, the most immediate means of doing so is to close the curtains (A). Although this might have been an accidental omission, the importance of privacy should be reiterated if the student nurse seems unclear (C). Patient choice is important, but other patients and visitors to the ward need to be considered as well. You can ask the patient before closing the curtains (B) but should probably do so regardless of his reply. You should always act on concerns regardless of whether you are directly involved in this staff–patient interaction (E). However, you should not embarrass colleagues or patients by reprimanding anyone in a manner which is unprofessional (D).

24. A, E, D, C, B

It is important that patients have an opportunity to answer questions, particularly about such an important issue. In this case, you should indicate to the patient that you will come back to answer questions (A). This is preferable to simply going back later (E) as it will reassure the patient to know there will be an additional opportunity. Although an in-depth explanation is necessary, you are an important part of the ward round whose absence might disrupt the care of other patients (D). You should not guarantee that the consultant will return as you are likely to have limited influence over his schedule (C). Insisting that the consultant remains at the bedside (B) would undermine his authority and potentially disrupt your working relationship.

25. B, C, A, D, E

You should take action as necessary to protect patient dignity. In this case, you should follow the patient to let him know that he is undressed (B) before helping tie the gown correctly (C). Shouting at the patient (A) would draw his attention but might also cause embarrassment. You could find a nurse to help, but this would distract a colleague from their role and would and miss the opportunity to act swiftly (D). Reprimanding the patient would be inappropriate as the gown is likely to be left untied in error (E).

26. D, C, E, B, A

Mittens risk causing patients significant distress and should only be used in limited circumstances. Most Trusts have strict criteria and rules for their use: the patient should either consent or lack capacity; the patient has pulled out lines; alternative strategies (e.g. distraction) have been unsuccessful (D). A patient without capacity at risk of pulling out lines (C) is a weaker candidate for mittens. Although imposing mittens is a clinical decision, next of kin should usually be supportive of their use (E). Otherwise, alternatives must be considered (e.g. one-to-one nursing) or the decision escalated to seniors. Absence of capacity (B) or confusion (A) are not in themselves good reasons for using mittens.

27. A, B, D, C, E

You should explore reasons for non-compliance (A) as the patient might be amenable to persuasion. It is important that the patient understands reasons for the restrictions (B) and that you have a legal duty to pass details of his condition to external authorities (D). Although ideally his GP should be informed, communication with the Health Protection Agency is a legal duty which must not be ignored (C). Discharging the patient from hospital without treatment (E) would put him and others at considerable risk from untreated tuberculosis. Another option must be found.

28. C, A, D, B, E

Ron may cause himself considerable harm by inadvertently pulling out lines and tubes. You should ensure Ron's safety using the minimum amount of restrictions. It might be possible to secure lines with bandages (C) or by placing them elsewhere (A). A one-to-one nurse can sometimes be arranged for short periods of time (D) when patients are at sufficient risk, although this depends on staffing arrangements. Mittens should only be used as a last resort when other strategies have failed and according to Trust policy (B). Taping pads to Ron's hands would be undignified and uncomfortable, and may worsen his agitation (E). If hands must be constrained, specially designed mittens should be used according to policy.

29. A, B, D, E, C

Sedation should only be prescribed when it is in your patient's interests. The interests of colleagues and other patients are secondary in this case. Although Ivy has severe dementia, you should try explaining that she is unsafe to mobilize (A). Other alternatives to sedation must be explored, such as distraction (B) or one-to-one nursing (D). When Ivy becomes particularly agitated and a risk to herself, sedation may be considered (E) regardless of consent. Prescribing PRN sedation should be avoided (C) as there is a risk of patients being over-sedated by nursing staff.

30. B, A, E, D, C

Patient care must be prioritized above educational commitments. You should first ask Rose whether you can examine her and that she would need to be in bed for this purpose (B). The nursing staff could set about hoisting Rose while you continue with your ward round (A).

Assessing Rose after your meeting (C) risks leaving her in discomfort for this period and potentially missing serious pathology. The latter is also a risk of inadequately examining your patient (D). Therefore you should miss the meeting if necessary because of this complication (E).

31. D, E, H

Competent adults can refuse any treatment, including cannulation. However, you have a duty to ensure that they understand the reason it is necessary and the likely consequences of refusal (E). This might be an appropriate time to consider converting to oral antibiotics (H) or a compromise might be necessary, such as offering to seek help from a colleague after another attempt (D). You should not accept Flora's refusal of further attempts without clear discussion of the need for intravenous antibiotics (C). This discussion should be realistic and not calculated to coerce the patient (A). You cannot guarantee that the next attempt will be successful (F) and there is no reason to think that Flora does not have capacity (G). Antibiotics should not be stopped in their entirety (B) simply because Flora is declining cannulation—oral equivalents may confer some benefit.

32. B, E, F

Compromise is always preferable and can only be achieved by understanding Randhir's concerns (B) and clarifying any misunderstandings (E). Regardless of conflict persisting, the discharge should be managed like any other with effective analgesia and follow-up (F). You should not make unhelpful statements, for example that nothing can be done to help (H) or that the bed is needed for 'more urgent' cases (D).

You should never mislead your consultant over which patients are under their care (A). It is unlikely that you can guarantee the timescale on which outpatient appointments are made (C). Regular strong opiate analgesia may be unhelpful if this cannot be continued in the community (G). This strategy should only be considered on specialist advice.

33. A, D, F

It is important not to let feelings cloud your professional judgement. The concern here is that Archie has become confused, which might be apparent objectively on calculating his AMTS (A). Otherwise unexplained personality changes warrant a full history, examination (F), and septic screen (D).

Your personal feelings should not cause you to move on prematurely (B) (H) or avoid seeing Archie (E) the following day. Documenting that Archie is a 'difficult patient' (C) adds little to his care. Conspiring to promote an early discharge is also unhelpful if Archie's personality change is the result of a pathological event (G).

34. B, E, G

Although formal confirmation of death should be done promptly, other considerations may be prioritized. The relatives may appreciate some time with the patient after which you should introduce yourself (E) and explain what the process involves (B). You should let the relatives choose whether to vacate the room (G) as some aspects (e.g. checking for pupillary reflexes) might distress them.

There is no need to ask for identification (D), make trite comments which may cause offence (F), or commence chest compressions (H) if there is a valid 'do not resuscitate' instruction. Financial (A) and bed management considerations (C) have no place at this time.

35. A, C, E

Any decisions about behaviour on the ward should be made in collaboration with the nursing staff (A). If it is agreed that Mike can administer his own methadone, he must be familiar with the equipment and safety requirements (C), and supervised (E) to ensure that sharps are appropriately discarded.

It would be inadvisable to alter Mike's regimen (D) without specialist advice or to give him needles (G) without addressing the issues above. Patients are often allowed to administer their own medication (B) (e.g. self-injecting insulin) when this is agreed with the nursing staff.

Hepatitis C emphasizes the importance of disposing of sharps safely but does not alter whether the process of self-injecting is permissible (F). Doctors should not usually accept the dose of methadone which someone who is drug-dependent has said they are usually prescribed (H). Independent verification is necessary (e.g. from a GP or pharmacy).

36. A, E, F

Doctors must advocate appropriately for their patients. If the wait is unusual, you should contact the rehabilitation hospital to check that Roger has not been missed (E). You should keep Roger informed (F) and ask the ward physiotherapists to do their best to mitigate the disadvantage of remaining in an acute hospital bed (A).

However, you should be sensitive to the resource allocations of other healthcare providers. Asking Roger's family to campaign (H) at the expense of other patients or insisting that the rehabilitation hospital find a bed (C) may be unhelpful. Daily inflammatory markers are inappropriate in a 'well' patient (B), but low molecular weight heparin should probably continue as his mobility is impaired (D). Discharge would only be appropriate if the multi-disciplinary team agree that Roger has returned to baseline and no longer requires prolonged rehabilitation (G).

37. C, F, H

Tom has a legal duty to inform the DVLA. Although this legal duty does not extend to doctors, you have a professional duty to balance the need for confidentiality against harm occurring to others. Therefore you cannot conspire with Tom to keep his driving secret (D).

You should ensure that Tom is fully informed about the risk of a second seizure (F) and that this advice is documented carefully (C). Your professional duty probably requires informing the DVLA if Tom refuses (H), but this should be made clear to him (E). Although it could be justifiable to inform Tom's employer, this is a more radical step and probably unnecessary if the DVLA is notified (B) (A). The hospital has no role to play in confiscating Tom's driving licence (G).

38. B, C, F

There is no obvious reason why Mark should wear a hospital gown (B) (A) and he certainly cannot be forced to wear one. Similarly, there is no clinical reason why Mark should be confined to hospital food (C). However, if this is having a negative impact on other patients, it may be worth bringing this to Mark's attention (F). Although the Ward Sister might want to talk to Mark, there is no reason why you shouldn't do so (H).

It cannot be assumed that all patients have people willing to bring them food (E) and neither does it follow that Mark must be fit enough for discharge (D). Moving Mark to a side room is a possibility, but only if one is available. He should certainly not be swapped for a patient isolated for clinical reasons (e.g. diarrhoea and vomiting) (G).

39. A, F, G

Although the patient has a GCS of 8, it is impossible to know to what extent he is aware of his surroundings. Therefore you should assume that he can hear and understand. You should explain the procedure fully (A) (G) and give warnings when appropriate (F).

You should not treat John differently because he is unresponsive, for example by careless attempts at cannulation (B), omission of important steps (E), or delegating the task inappropriately (C). John is a vulnerable patient as he cannot advocate for himself and so his care should not be deferred until later (D). Giving oral fluid to an unresponsive patient is likely to result in aspiration (H).

40. C, D, G

In this scenario you must balance the dignity and comfort of one patient against the need to take a second blood sample from another. You should certainly help the patient on the commode if you are able (C) or ask a nurse to do so (D). Clearly, it is not appropriate for a patient to be left on the commode shouting and it is likely the nurses are occupied elsewhere. You could apologize for this without the need to assign blame (G). Clearly, reprimanding the patient for shouting is not helpful (H).

Letting the patient know that you are in a hurry is only helpful if it precedes your assurance that someone else will help shortly (A) (B). A vague reassurance that 'someone' will 'probably' help soon is unhelpful (E). The patient should not be encouraged to abuse their emergency bell (F).

Working effectively as part of a team

Introduction

Questions within this section highlight your ability and willingness to work with team members. You will need to work collaboratively and respectfully within a multi-disciplinary team, as well as provide advice and support to colleagues. A willingness to take on more responsibility must always be balanced by an openness to share your workload when necessary.

You should always favour a collaborative approach when answering SJT questions, and part of this domain requires an understanding of your role and the role of others. Recognizing skills and qualities allows you to adapt and demonstrate leadership by utilizing the skills of appropriate individuals to achieve specific goals.

- Different individuals and professions will bring unique perspectives which might result in conflict. Understand what each person is trying to achieve; and remember that you all share the goal of making patients better.
- Respect the fact that other team members have multiple demands on their time. Only they can truly know the extent of their workload.
- Try to resolve conflict with the individuals concerned before escalating issues unnecessarily. When an issue arises with a non-doctor, this might best be resolved using their own hierarchy. The nursing staff, including healthcare assistants (HCAs), are supervised by a Ward Sister who will often answer to a Matron.

QUESTIONS

1. A porter tells you that he has seen an HCA take something from a patient's personal belongings.

*Rank in order the following actions in response to this situation
(1 = Most appropriate; 5 = Least appropriate)*

A Ask the HCA to open her locker and empty her pockets.

B Establish exactly what the porter has seen, and confirm with the patient that they have something missing before informing the Ward Sister.

C Call the police.

D Ask the porter to find out more by speaking to the patient and HCA.

E Report the incident to your consultant.

2. You are on a renal medicine ward round and notice your consultant lose his balance but quickly correct himself. You find his behaviour slightly unusual and can smell alcohol on his breath. Although the decisions he is making appear appropriate, you wonder if he has been drinking alcohol earlier in the day.

*Rank in order the following actions in response to this situation
(1 = Most appropriate; 5 = Least appropriate)*

A Ask the consultant whether he has been drinking alcohol.

B Speak to the consultant's secretary about his behaviour.

C Discuss your concerns with your registrar and ask whether he feels that the consultant is acting out of character.

D Inform the Clinical Director.

E Speak with the consultant, and share your concerns about what you think you have seen recently.

3. You have asked a nurse to administer a heparin infusion. On returning to the ward three hours later you find that the infusion has still not been given as the nurse has been busy with other tasks.

*Rank in order the following actions in response to this situation
(1 = Most appropriate; 5 = Least appropriate)*

A Explain the urgency of giving the heparin, and ask her to prepare the infusion straight away.

B Avoid antagonizing the nurse by leaving her to complete her jobs.

C Speak to the nurse in charge about the delay.

D Confront the nurse on the ward and insist that she prepares the infusion straight away.

E Go to the preparation room and prepare the heparin infusion yourself.

4. It is your first day on the neurology ward and all junior doctors are changing jobs. You are asked by the ward clerk to complete a discharge summary for a patient who was discharged last week, including arrangements for follow-up.

Rank in order the following actions in response to this situation (1 = Most appropriate; 5 = Least appropriate)

A Refuse and ask the ward clerk to find the foundation doctor who was looking after the patient.

B Ask the new SHO to try and complete it.

C Attempt to complete the TTO ([medicines] to take out) and try to find the consultant and ask them about follow-up arrangements.

D Write a letter to the previous junior doctor for the neurology ward and ask them to complete the TTO for their patient.

E Complete the TTO to the best of your ability and arrange routine clinic follow-up in six weeks.

5. A patient approaches you to say that she overheard your registrar swearing repeatedly when he was at the nursing station. She does not wish to make a formal complaint at the moment, but suggests that you do something about his language.

Rank in order the following actions in response to this situation (1 = Most appropriate; 5 = Least appropriate)

A Raise the concern privately with your registrar.

B Inform PALS.

C Apologize to the patient and assure her that you will speak to the doctor involved.

D Establish what exactly was said and when.

E Explain that the registrar is 'only human' and that she should not listen to conversations at the nursing station as they might be confidential.

6. You are working with Dr Green, a GP, about whom you are concerned because he never seems to examine his patients. He appears willing to refer some patients and send others home without as much as a basic physical examination. However, he is well liked by his patients and colleagues, and he has never been subject to a complaint or any disciplinary action.

Choose the THREE most appropriate actions to take in this situation

A You have no substantial proof of malpractice and therefore cannot report your concerns at the moment.

B The collective support of Dr Green at the practice should dissuade you from making a complaint.

C Telephone the GMC to raise your concerns with them.

D Ask the GP about his decisions not to examine patients.

E Attempt to discuss the issue privately with other colleagues at the practice.

F Inform the Primary Care Trust.

G Contact your Educational Supervisor.

H Inform the British Medical Association.

7. Your registrar inadvertently prescribes a ten times dose of methotrexate which you spot before the first dose is given. The registrar breathes a sigh of relief that the error was spotted and tells you both he and the patient had a 'lucky escape'.

Rank in order the following actions in response to this situation
(1 = Most appropriate; 5 = Least appropriate)

A Agree that you are lucky as well, as you would have to complete a long clinical incident form if it had been administered.

B Raise the issue with the nursing staff so that they are aware of common mistakes to look out for.

C Mention the prescribing error to the lead pharmacist.

D Raise the issue with your consultant at the next ward round.

E Complete a formal incident report.

8. At a multi-disciplinary team meeting, a nurse expresses concern about a patient's ability to mobilize safely at home. The occupational therapy team disagree and an argument ensues. Five minutes later they are continuing to argue, and no progress has been made.

Rank in order the following actions in response to this situation
(1 = Most appropriate; 5 = Least appropriate)

A Move the agenda onto the next patient, and return to the controversial case at the end.

B Ask the nurse to elaborate on her concerns.

C Ask the occupational therapist to leave the meeting.

D Invite the social worker to share her opinion.

E Do not become involved.

9. You are an FY1 in orthopaedics. You have found the physiotherapist to be particularly challenging to work with. She frequently ignores the postoperative plan for mobilizing patients and seems to actively discourage patients being discharged home. Your registrar says that the physiotherapist is 'obstructive'.

Rank in order the following actions in response to this situation
(1 = Most appropriate; 5 = Least appropriate)

A Speak to the other members of the multi-disciplinary team prior to weekly meetings to establish the discharge plan.

B Ask for the physiotherapist to be replaced.

C Invite the physiotherapist to join your consultant ward round so that discharge arrangements can be made face-to-face.

D Ask an impartial senior colleague for advice.

E Follow the physiotherapist's advice, as she is ultimately responsible for the patient's safe mobilization.

10. You have been working as the FY1 in the Medical Assessment Unit for two months. On many occasions during the rushed morning handover, you have found that tasks are not appropriately trans-ferred from the night doctors to the morning team. The ethos is focused on handing over quickly so that the night team can get home to sleep.

Rank in order the following actions in response to this situation (1 = Most appropriate; 5 = Least appropriate)

A Ensure that your own handover is effective.

B Arrange a meeting with your colleagues to explain your concerns.

C File incident reports for each individual whom you believe to be failing in their responsibilities.

D Only comment if urgent tasks are not handed over as it is not worth making a fuss over routine jobs.

E Inform the consultant in charge that handover arrangements are inadequate.

11. Frances, an FY1 colleague, confides in you that she was recently diagnosed with thyroid cancer. She does not appear to be symp-tomatic and is scheduled to undergo a biopsy and surgical treatment at another hospital in a month's time. Although she is not as spritely as usual, you have not noticed any change in her performance.

Rank in order the following actions in response to this situation (1 = Most appropriate; 5 = Least appropriate)

A Suggest that she refers herself for counselling via Occupational Health.

B Advise Frances to inform her Educational Supervisor.

C Inform your consultant immediately.

D Gently explore how she is feeling about the diagnosis.

E Keep an eye on Frances at work but do not say anything to anyone else.

12. Rachel, a fellow FY1, is a budding surgeon and frequently abandons the ward so that she can assist in theatre. Except for the morning ward round, you have not seen Rachel on the ward for at least five weeks. Your consultant appears content with this arrangement as long as the tasks are completed, and you do not have a particular interest in surgery.

Rank in order the following actions in response to this situation
(1 = Most appropriate; 5 = Least appropriate)

A Do nothing as you enjoy the ward and Rachel clearly wants to be in theatre.

B Speak to Rachel and insist that she spends more time on the ward.

C Go to theatre and leave any ward jobs until after hours when both you and Rachel can attend to them.

D Suggest that FY1s should be prohibited from going to theatre until all ward jobs are completed.

E Talk to Rachel and suggest dividing theatre and ward time more evenly.

13. You overhear a medical student on the bus who is giving a rather unfavourable description of your consultant's clinical competence. You do not believe that it is his intention to be deliberately heard, but it is clear that other passengers are listening.

Rank in order the following actions in response to this situation
(1 = Most appropriate; 5 = Least appropriate)

A Explain that the student might have misunderstood the reasons for the consultant's decision.

B Do nothing as it is a public place and medical students are not Trust employees.

C Try to catch the medical student another day to explain that his comments were unhelpful.

D Write a letter to the dean of his medical school.

E Suggest to the student that he exercises caution when talking about colleagues in public.

14. Your registrar frequently undermines your organizational skills on the morning ward round. He expects you to take what you believe is unfair initiative in terms of organizing investigations before the patients are reviewed by a senior member of the team. He also criticizes your note writing and you cannot seem to avoid this, whatever changes you make to your documentation style.

Rank in order the following actions in response to this situation
(1 = Most appropriate; 5 = Least appropriate)

A Explain to the registrar privately that you feel that he expects too much initiative from an FY1.

B Ask the registrar to show you how he would like notes taken on the ward round.

C Inform your consultant that the registrar is constantly belittling your abilities as a doctor.

D Arrange a meeting with Medical Staffing and ask that you are timetabled so as to avoid the registrar as much as possible.

E Ignore your registrar's interpersonal style but try to accommodate his whims.

15. Each time you phone radiology, you receive a barrage of criticism from a particularly discourteous radiology registrar. Your colleagues now try to make fewer requests whenever this particular registrar is on duty. He once criticized your 'incoherent' radiology requests and, when you asked how your requests could be improved, he hung up the phone.

Rank in order the following actions in response to this situation
(1 = Most appropriate; 5 = Least appropriate)

A Arrange a meeting between the radiology registrar and the Mess President.

B Raise the issue with your Clinical Supervisor.

C Ask for a slot at the monthly radiology meeting to discuss communication between junior doctors and duty registrars.

D Contact the Clinical Director for Radiology to explain your difficulty.

E Avoid making radiology requests when this registrar is on duty unless they are absolutely necessary.

16. Your SHO discloses to you that she is going through a very difficult separation and occasionally has suicidal thoughts.

Choose the THREE most appropriate actions to take in this situation

A Reassure her and tell her that everything will be OK.

B Do not get involved with her personal affairs.

C Offer a friendly ear if and when she wishes to talk further.

D Suggest that she attends counselling.

E Suggest that she books an appointment with her GP.

F Suggest that she speaks to her Educational Supervisor.

G Ask the registrar to prescribe antidepressants.

17. You are reviewing your patients on the ward round, and Mrs Egbert asks if you will need to perform another examination 'down below' as it was uncomfortable yesterday. You cannot understand why this was performed during the SHO's ward round, and the examination had not been detailed in the medical notes.

Choose the THREE most appropriate actions to take in this situation

A Inform the vulnerable adults' nurse.

B Inform your consultant.

C Attempt to establish more detail about Mrs Egbert's complaints and the nature of the examination.

D Ask your SHO to describe his review of Mrs Egbert yesterday.

E Speak to the SHO in front of the registrar at the evening handover.

F Contact your Medical Director.

G Inform the patient's family about what has happened.

H Ask the patient not to reveal any information about the incident to anyone else until her consultant has spoken to her.

18. Despite your best efforts, your Educational Supervisor refuses to see you because he is too busy. Eight weeks into your rotation, he eventually asks you to attend theatre and tries to complete your induction meeting between surgical cases, but only manages to spend a few minutes talking to you. He concludes your brief encounter by asking you to sign an online educational agreement.

Choose the THREE most appropriate actions to take in this situation

A Sign the agreement, and go home and read it in more detail.

B Do not sign the educational agreement.

C Establish whether it will be possible to arrange a more effective meeting in the near future.

D Ask your Educational Supervisor to arrange for a suitable replacement.

E Ask your Clinical Supervisor to act as your Educational Supervisor instead.

F Report your Educational Supervisor to the deanery.

G Arrange a meeting with the Foundation Programme Director.

H Persist with future brief meetings.

19. Your registrar asks you to prepare a presentation for the hospital grand round. You are very keen to present at the grand round, although eventually you realize that she intends to present the case in its entirety and merely wants you to do the preparation work.

Rank in order the following actions in response to this situation
(1 = Most appropriate; 5 = Least appropriate)

A Ask the registrar if you can present at least part of the case, as it will be good experience.

B Ask the registrar to make a case presentation for you to present the following week.

C Inform your consultant about your registrar's lack of fairness.

D Refuse to hand over the slides for the presentation.

E Do nothing as she is your senior and there has been educational value in producing the slides.

20. Your registrar suffers from reflux disease and is experiencing very bad heartburn after lunch. His symptoms stop him from carrying out the ward round. He informs a nurse he forgot to take his usual proton pump inhibitor that morning and is given omeprazole from the drug cabinet.

Rank in order the following actions in response to this situation
(1 = Most appropriate; 5 = Least appropriate)

A Report the registrar for taking patient medication.

B Suggest that he obtains the medication from A&E by admitting himself as a patient and having the medicine formally prescribed.

C Offer to prescribe omeprazole for your registrar on a discharge summary prescription.

D Reprimand the nurse who has given him the PPI.

E Do nothing.

21. You overhear a conversation between two of your foundation colleagues, Peter and James. Peter describes receiving a police caution the previous weekend during a raucous outing that followed a stressful week of on-call nights. The nature of the offence sounds fairly benign, but it does not seem as if your colleague has any intention of informing anybody else.

Rank in order the following actions in response to this situation
(1 = Most appropriate; 5 = Least appropriate)

A Tell Peter that you will be informing the GMC.

B Arrange a meeting with Peter's Educational Supervisor to discuss what you heard.

C Speak to Peter about what you have heard, and whether he is aware of the guidance related to receiving cautions.

D Do nothing as the offence sounds relatively benign and no harm has been done.

E Speak to James, and establish more details about the nature of the events.

22. You learn that your colleague is struggling to cannulate patients, despite being in his second FY1 placement.

Rank in order the following actions in response to this situation
(1 = Most appropriate; 5 = Least appropriate)

A Help to train your colleague by guiding him through cannulation, and practising in the clinical skills laboratory.

B Ignore the problem unless a serious incident occurs.

C Tell your colleague to ask a senior for help.

D Fastbleep the consultant in order to share your concerns with him.

E Email his Clinical Supervisor.

23. You are assisting a senior registrar in theatre during an inguinal hernia repair. You have seen a lot of hernia repairs during your training, and you are certain that the registrar has inadvertently tied off the vas deferens during this operation. Your registrar denies this but, when you ask him to identify the vas, he does not respond convincingly.

Rank in order the following actions in response to this situation
(1 = Most appropriate; 5 = Least appropriate)

A Accept that your registrar is much more experienced and probably correct.

B Ask the anaesthetist to become involved.

C Allow the procedure to be completed before raising the issue with the consultant in charge.

D Insist that the surgeon stops as you are confident that a mistake has been made.

E Leave the operating table and contact the consultant, asking him to attend the theatre.

24. Jill is a specialist nurse on your renal team. She is very knowledgeable, but you feel that she can be overbearing in clinical situations and you frequently feel undermined in your position as a junior doctor.

Choose the THREE most appropriate actions to take in this situation

A Discuss your feelings with Jill and ask how she thinks you could overcome this difficulty.

B Remind Jill of your superior position as a doctor.

C Adopt a more confident approach to patient care.

D Try to gain Jill's respect by finding an opportunity to challenge her clinical judgement and demonstrate your superior knowledge.

E Adopt a more subordinate position as you are less experienced.

F Speak to your senior colleagues for advice.

G Ask the nursing staff whether they find Jill difficult to work with.

H Do nothing as long as her behaviour does not impact on clinical care.

25. Annabelle, the Ward Sister, has bleeped you and asks you to prescribe atenolol to a patient who is hypertensive. After reviewing the patient, you disagree and feel that anti-hypertensives are not clinically indicated. Annabelle is not convinced by your explanation, saying that in her 'extensive experience' they are needed.

Rank in order the following actions in response to this situation (1 = Most appropriate; 5 = Least appropriate)

A Explain how and why you arrived at your decision not to prescribe anti-hypertensives.

B Insist on your management plan as you are responsible for signing the prescription.

C Agree to prescribe anti-hypertensives, but ask the patient's GP to stop them on discharge.

D Inform Annabelle that you will discuss the issue with a senior colleague, but that she should not give any medication for the time being.

E Agree that she should give the medication but do not sign the prescription chart.

26. Vera is an elderly patient on the orthogeriatrics ward who is currently receiving 20 minutes of counselling a week from the psychologist. After reviewing her, you believe that she might benefit from more regular counselling.

Rank in order the following actions in response to this situation (1 = Most appropriate; 5 = Least appropriate)

A Speak to other multi-disciplinary team members before the weekly meeting to gauge their thoughts.

B Invite Vera and her family to the multi-disciplinary team meeting to voice their concerns.

C Continue with the psychologist's current treatment plan.

D Tell the psychologist he should visit Vera at least twice a week.

E Ask the psychologist whether they think Vera might benefit from additional input.

27. There is a cardiac arrest call in the outpatients clinic at the other side of the hospital. You arrive to find a nurse performing chest compressions being watched by a domestic assistant and a final-year medical student.

Rank in order the following actions in response to this situation
(1 = Most appropriate; 5 = Least appropriate)

A Instruct the medical student to take over chest compressions.

B Encourage the medical student to lead the crash call to develop his leadership skills.

C Instruct the domestic assistant to bring the crash trolley.

D Instruct the medical student to bring the crash trolley, while you take over chest compressions.

E Wait for instructions from the nurse doing compressions.

28. You are planning to review all your patients quickly before the consultant's weekly ward round. The pharmacist insists that you immediately change all your 'as required' prescriptions of paracetamol from '1g qds' to '500mg—1g qds' according to a new Trust guideline. She says that she will have to call your consultant if you don't do this immediately. You have no concerns about your original prescription, and there are 25 patients for whom this would need to be rewritten.

Rank in order the following actions in response to this situation
(1 = Most appropriate; 5 = Least appropriate)

A Tell the pharmacist to call your consultant as you have other tasks to complete before the ward round.

B Explain to the pharmacist that there is no substantial difference between the prescriptions but that you will speak to your consultant when he begins the ward round.

C Tell the pharmacist that you will correct your prescription charts immediately.

D Tell the pharmacist that you will return after the ward round if possible to complete the task.

E Tell the pharmacist that you will hand this over to the evening team.

29. You are working on a busy surgical on-call shift when you are bleeped for a fifth time by a junior nurse for another 'trivial' task which could wait until the regular team arrives the following day.

Rank in order the following actions in response to this situation
(1 = Most appropriate; 5 = Least appropriate)

A Tell her not to phone you again.

B Explain how few doctors are working out of hours and how to decide which jobs require urgent attention.

C Go to the ward and ask the senior nurse to triage all further bleeps.

D Take the referral and add it to your list of tasks.

E Listen to the referral while asking for appropriate details.

30. You are confident that your patient requires an abdominal ultrasound scan but the radiologist has refused your request twice, initially because of insufficient clinical details, and then for unconvincing blood results. Your consultant has insisted that the scan is done today.

Rank in order the following actions in response to this situation
(1 = Most appropriate; 5 = Least appropriate)

A Speak to another radiologist.

B Explain that your consultant has examined the patient and, unless the radiologist is willing to do the same, he should accept the request.

C Ask your consultant for advice.

D Take the medical notes and go to speak with the radiologist in person.

E Do not order the ultrasound scan.

31. While working as the surgical FY1 over the weekend, you are asked to complete a discharge letter for a patient whom you have never met. After searching his medical notes, you are unable to find any clear plan for follow-up. The Ward Sister is unsure, and the registrar is in emergency theatre. The patient and his family are insistent on leaving as they have waited more than four hours for his discharge letter.

Choose the THREE most appropriate actions to take in this situation

A Keep trying to contact your surgical registrar.

B Apologize for the delay and explain you have been seeing unwell patients for the last few hours.

C Ask the patient to telephone the consultant's secretary in two weeks if he has not received a follow-up appointment.

D Book a routine postoperative clinic appointment with the consultant in six weeks.

E Leave a clear note for the attention of the surgical team asking them to contact the patient to arrange further follow-up.

F Ask the GP to decide the follow-up.

G Ask the medical registrar for advice.

H Ask the patient to sign a disclaimer stating he is leaving against medical advice.

32. You are trying to arrange two weeks of annual leave in six months time to attend your friend's wedding abroad. Despite emailing and telephoning the rota coordinator at the hospital where you will be working, you have been unable to secure the time away.

Choose the THREE most appropriate actions to take in this situation

A Write a formal letter of complaint to the hospital.

B Try to arrange cover by swapping your annual leave with a colleague once the rota is published.

C Inform your future Clinical Supervisor that you will be requesting annual leave.

D Send a further email to the rota coordinator, copying in anyone else who might be able to help, such as the Human Resources representative looking after new foundation doctors.

E Contact a locum agency to assess the cost and availability of cover.

F Do not make any further attempts to arrange your leave for fear of antagonizing the rota coordinator.

G Cancel your plans to attend the wedding.

H Inform your current Clinical Supervisor.

33. After the afternoon surgical ward round, you have amassed a long list of tasks. These include seven venepunctures and an outpatient venesection which was scheduled for an hour ago, two cannulas, and three discharge summaries. You consider how you will complete these tasks.

Rank in order the following actions in response to this situation
(1 = Most appropriate; 5 = Least appropriate)

A Bleep the phlebotomy team to ask for assistance while you approach the outpatient venesection.

B Attend the outpatient department where you were scheduled to perform a venesection an hour ago, and then prioritize the other tasks.

C Hand over your list of jobs to the ward nurse and ask her to bleep you if there are any problems.

D Head to the coffee shop with FY1 friends to prioritize your tasks and recruit help if possible.

E Ask another FY1 for help.

34. As the FY1 in gastroenterology, you are arranging the discharge of a patient who is dependent on alcohol and was admitted with symptoms of withdrawal. He has many social problems, including unemployment and long-term disability. In an effort to maintain abstinence from alcohol, you consider the different healthcare professionals you will need to involve, as well as outpatient follow-up with your consultant.

Choose the THREE most appropriate actions to take in this situation

A Ward Sister working on the admitting ward.

B General practitioner.

C Drug and alcohol liaison officer.

D Housing assistant.

E Social worker.

F Citizen's Advice Bureau.

G Psychologist.

H Liver transplant services.

35. You are coming to the end of your first FY1 rotation in endocrinology. The job was challenging and you felt inadequately prepared for many of the responsibilities during induction. You consider how you might go about helping your successor.

Rank in order the following actions in response to this situation
(1 = Most appropriate; 5 = Least appropriate)

A Feed back your thoughts on the induction to your Clinical Supervisor during your final meeting.

B Write a list of useful tips for your successor.

C Take a week off your next rotation to help support your successor during their first week.

D Leave your mobile phone number for your successor to contact you if they encounter difficulties.

E Leave the induction process to the Foundation Programme management team.

36. Your SHO has a habit of sending text messages on his phone during the ward round. Your consultant has not noticed, but you have seen a number of patients and relatives appear less than impressed with his inattention.

Rank in order the following actions in response to this situation
(1 = Most appropriate; 5 = Least appropriate)

A Let the SHO know that others have noticed him sending text messages.

B Ask the SHO whether everything is OK.

C Suggest that the SHO put his phone away immediately.

D Inform the consultant.

E Initiate a 'politeness code', including a rule against excessive texting, which all members of the team should sign.

37. You are working on a busy medical ward which is famously understaffed. Since your new SHO started the rotation two weeks ago, she has left work 45 minutes early every day to collect her children from school. You are working until 8 p.m. most days and still feel that you are not on top of the workload.

Rank in order the following actions in response to this situation
(1 = Most appropriate; 5 = Least appropriate)

A Ask her to cover you for the first 45 minutes of your shift.

B Ask her to work during her lunch break to make up the missing time.

C Arrange a meeting with your consultant to discuss her early departure.

D Tell the SHO that you will be informing the consultant unless she is able to make alternative arrangements for the collection of her children.

E Establish whether the childcare arrangements are temporary.

38. Your registrar is known for his strong opinions. As an aside from the ward round, he tells the group of juniors that migrants from Eastern Europe are stretching the NHS to breaking point. You are aware of a Polish patient nearby who is listening intently and appears to be taking offence.

Choose the THREE most appropriate actions to take in this situation

A Apologize to the patient for your registrar's comments.

B Try to move the ward round on to the next patient.

C Challenge the registrar's viewpoint by outlining the contribution immigrants have made to the NHS.

D Agree with the registrar to appease him and move the ward round on.

E Speak to the registrar privately after the ward round about how you felt that the patient was reacting.

F Leave the round to speak to the consultant.

G Share your concerns with the consultant if your registrar does not become more sensitive.

H Return to the patient after the ward round to suggest that they make a formal complaint.

39. A fellow FY1 regularly takes home surgical supplies (e.g. disposable tools and sutures) to practise surgical skills.

Rank in order the following actions in response to this situation
(1 = Most appropriate; 5 = Least appropriate)

A Speak to the theatre manager about equipment being taken inappropriately.

B Insist that if your colleague continues to take hospital property you will have to report him.

C Email his Clinical Supervisor with the details.

D Do nothing as it is good that your colleague is practising to become a better doctor.

E Insist that he returns the hospital property immediately.

40. It is the third consecutive week that your SHO has not covered your duties in the preoperative assessment clinic for an hour whilst you attend mandatory teaching. Each time she has arrived 30 minutes late, despite being given plenty of warning. She always says she has been busy with the ward patients.

Choose the THREE most appropriate actions to take in this situation

A Leave the preoperative assessment clinic with instructions that the SHO should be bleeped if she does not arrive.

B Bleep the registrar and ask her to contact the SHO before each teaching session.

C Inform your consultant that you are not meeting teaching commitments because there is inadequate cover for your absence.

D Ask a colleague to sign you into the teaching and pick up an extra handout.

E Speak to your SHO to identify what is stopping her from arriving and whether her tasks can be re-prioritized.

F Email the teaching coordinator to explain your absence.

G Arrange for the nurse specialist to cover your duties for the hour during teaching.

H Ask the clinical secretaries to shorten the preoperative assessment clinics by an hour.

ANSWERS

1. B, E, D, A, C

All healthcare professionals are in positions of trust and must act within the highest standards of integrity. The porter has made a very serious allegation which could have damaging legal and professional consequences. For this reason, the initial claim justifies some preliminary investigation to broadly establish the facts (B) before informing the Ward Sister. The Ward Sister is a more practical and appropriate port of call than your consultant (E), particularly as she is responsible for the nurses and HCAs on the ward. It is not the responsibility of the porter to gather more evidence (D) and it is not your place to ask a colleague to open her locker and empty her pockets (A). Although it mah be necessary to call the police, this is likely to be handled by hospital security who will have more experience of dealing with similar issues (C).

2. E, A, D, C, B

It is essential to ensure the safety of patients. You should first explain your concerns privately (E) and ascertain whether your consultant may be under the influence of alcohol (A).

If this is admitted or you are not convinced by his denial, you should ensure that he leaves the clinical area. This should be done discreetly but involving other staff and/or security if necessary. Once the situation has been made safe, you have a duty to report the incident to an appropriate person, in this case the Clinical Director (D). Involving other members of staff (C) (B) would only be justifiable if you are insufficiently certain to approach your consultant directly. If your concern is justifiable and genuinely held, you should involve as few colleagues as possible to minimize professional embarrassment.

3. A, C, E, D, B

Effective working relationships require individuals to have some discretion about planning their workload. However, the nurse may not appreciate the urgency of the task and this should be reiterated (A). If a further delay is anticipated, it may be necessary to escalate the issue as the nurse in charge (C) might intervene or to allocate a nurse from elsewhere to help. If the nursing staff are genuinely too busy and you are happy to prepare the infusion yourself, you could do so (E). However, this is only an option if you can perform this task safely. Although the infusion needs to be administered, insisting that it is done immediately is unlikely to help foster a positive working relationship (D). It might be ineffective and risks harming the likelihood of other tasks being completed in a timely manner. However, you must advocate for your patient and it is not sufficient to satisfy yourself that a drug was prescribed if you know that it has not been administered (B).

4. C, E, B, D, A

Ideally, discharge summaries should ideally be completed by a involved in the patient's care. However, if the outgoing team neglected to complete one, it is important that it is completed to the best of your ability. As you are unfamiliar with the patient and local policy for follow-up, you should check with a senior colleague who might remember the case (C). Although not ideal, arranging a routine appointment in six weeks would ensure that the patient is not lost to follow-up (E). You could ask your SHO to complete the task, but they have also rotated posts and are unlikely to add anything further to the discharge summary (B). Although courtesy requires completing routine tasks before rotating to a new job, it would be inappropriate to expect your predecessor to complete the discharge summary when they are now in a new post and/or hospital (D) (A).

5. D, C, A, E, B

Doctors have a duty to act professionally at all times and it would seem that your registrar might have erred in this respect. You should gather preliminary facts (D) before reassuring the patient that you will raise her concerns, even if she does not wish to make a formal complaint (C). You should then speak privately to the registrar so that he is aware of the concerns (A). Reprimanding the patient would be unfair and might either precipitate a formal complaint or reduce the likelihood of her raising concerns in future (E). Informing PALS would be inappropriate, although the patient might wish to explore this option if she is dissatisfied with your response (B).

6. D, E, G

If you have concerns with the standard of care given to patients, you have a duty to report them, particularly if patients are potentially at risk. You should not be dissuaded from raising concerns because a doctor is popular (B) or you do not have proof (A). Ideally, concerns of this nature should be raised with the doctor involved in the first instance (D). He might explain his decisions and/or modify his practice without further action being necessary. If advice is needed as to how to proceed, other senior colleagues (E) and/or your Educational Supervisor (G) are appropriate contacts.

Informing the Primary Care Trust (F) or the British Medical Association (H) would be inappropriate and, although a GMC referral might be necessary at some point (C), a concern of this nature might be more effectively dealt with informally.

7. E, C, D, B, A

Clinical incident reporting is important for identifying local error patterns. For this reason, a report should be completed for the 'near miss' even though the patient came to no harm (E) (A). Although it is probably not necessary to tell the lead pharmacist, they would at least direct you to complete an incident report if informed (C). Your consultant could be told (D) but is likely to be sent a copy of the incident report, and you do not wish to cause your registrar unnecessary professional embarrassment by raising the issue too often. Similarly, it would be unhelpful to inform the nursing staff (B) unless this was necessary to stop the dose being given once it has been crossed off the drug chart.

8. B, A, D, E, C

Multi-disciplinary team meetings are important forums for identifying and solving medical and social problems in conjunction with allied health professional colleagues. It is not necessarily the doctor's responsibility to lead such meetings, but you do have a shared responsibility to ensure that the team is working effectively. In this case, time is being wasted and you should help to facilitate the team arrive at a decision. You could suggest giving the nurse space to voice her concerns uninterrupted (B). Alternatively, it might be worth returning to the case later on so that it can be addressed with fresh minds and progress can be made through the agenda (A).

Although the social worker might have an opinion, she has not contributed so far and this might suggest that she has nothing specific to add (D). You could leave the nurse and occupational therapist to resolve their differences (E), but progress must be made eventually. It is not your place to ask anyone to leave the meeting (C), and this would be the wrong time to lose the occupational therapist's expertise.

9. D, C, A, B, E

Personality clashes and differences in approach are inevitable consequences of multi-disciplinary team working. However, these must not be allowed to impact on patient care. Although neither surgeons nor physiotherapists are necessarily 'correct' about optimal mobilization arrangements, consensus is more likely to follow collaborative working. A senior colleague might be able to suggest changes to local policies and protocols (D) which might include multi-disciplinary ward rounds (C). In the meantime, you could involve other members of the multi-disciplinary team (e.g. nurses and occupational therapists) in discharge arrangements so that a consensus is established before meetings take place (A).

Asking for the physiotherapist to be replaced (B) is likely to damage working relationships, and this is rarely the place of a junior doctor rotating temporarily through a post. You should not blindly accept the physiotherapist's advice when this conflicts with that of your consultant (E). Mobilization arrangements will depend on operative considerations (e.g. bone quality, fracture pattern, and choice of metalwork), details to which the physiotherapist may not have access. The consultant is ultimately responsible for patient care and should be informed if his instructions are routinely being disregarded.

10. B, E, A, C, D

Handover between teams must be done correctly to ensure that important tasks are not missed. This is particularly vital given current employment regulations which have shifted the job pattern of doctors to shift working.

As this issue relates to a group of doctors, you should assess the degree of support that you have for change and whether others have suggestions (B). You should then approach a senior colleague (E) to suggest changes, for example starting the handover meeting at an earlier time. Your own handover should be effective (A) but this might be hindered if there are adverse structural issues, such as other doctors wanting you to hurry up. In this case, the culture of accepting poor-quality handovers must be challenged. Submitting incident reports for many different doctors (C) will make you unpopular. Although it might result in change, it risks creating a personal issue out of a cultural problem and would not be a measured response to your problem. There is no such thing as a 'routine' task—either it needs to be done or it doesn't. Even checking a 'routine' blood test is important if the patient is found to be severely hyperkalaemic. Doing nothing (D) in this case is not an option.

11. D, B, E, A, C

You should be aware of factors which might cause colleagues to under-perform, including poor health. As Frances has confided in you, it would seem appropriate to ask how she feels (D) and whether she is coping. Ideally, she should let her Educational Supervisor know in case anything can be done, or must be done in future, to support her at work (B). However, unless there is a risk of Frances underperforming and putting patients at risk, informing others must be her choice. It is not your place to tell other people unless a serious concern is raised (C). Nevertheless, you might want to remain aware of how Frances is managing at work (E) in case other actions become appropriate later on. Although Frances may benefit from counselling, you cannot presume that this is something she would want (A).

12. E, B, D, A, C

As foundation doctors, both you and Rachel are expected to gain specific competencies. Rachel is at risk of not doing this effectively. Similarly, as an FY1 on a surgical placement, you should assist in theatre if there is time available, as this is also relevant experience. Although it is reasonable to divide tasks according to your respective interests, you should both aim to gain experience of each setting.

You should first talk to Rachel (E) as this is preferable to confronting her about being absent from the ward (B). Although you could agree informally, it should be unnecessary to establish a rule that FY1s can only assist in theatre at a set time (D). As the situation risks both you and Rachel missing out on important experience, it would be wrong to do nothing simply because you are comfortable (A). The only inappropriate option would be abandoning the ward yourself (C) without prior arrangement and leaving potentially important tasks until late in the day.

13. **E, A, C, B, D**

Your first step should be to stop the medical student continuing this conversation in public as colleagues (like patients) are entitled to a degree of privacy. You are most likely to stop the student by drawing his attention to the fact that he can be overheard (E) and indicating that the situation might have been misunderstood (A). Although you could catch him at another time (C), this would not stop further damage being inflicted on your consultant's reputation by the conversation continuing. Doing nothing would be unhelpful to the medical students (who need guidance), your consultant (who needs support in his absence), and other passengers (whose trust in the medical profession might be damaged) (B). Medical students are expected to exercise professionalism in the same way as doctors as they are privy to a similar set of privileged experiences. Although writing to the medical school dean might be necessary (depending on what was said), it does not seem to be a measured response to the circumstances (D).

14. **A, B, C, E, D**

Mutual respect is essential to any effective professional relationship. Your registrar might not realize how unconstructive his style has become and he might improve if approached directly (A). You should try to show willingness to improve by asking to be shown how he would like notes to be taken (B). This might also reduce confrontation in future. If the situation does not improve, you should certainly seek advice from your consultant in the first instance (C). Although you might be tempted simply to accommodate the registrar's whims (E), his caustic style is likely to be deployed against other colleagues, not all of whom will be as stoical. Therefore his interpersonal style should be addressed.

Although harassment should certainly be escalated, asking to be timetabled so as to avoid the registrar does not address the route cause (D). It is also likely to cause disruption to other team members and service commitments.

15. **B, D, C, E, A**

The NHS employs 1.4 million people, some of whom have challenging personalities. However, if junior doctors are dissuaded from requesting investigations because of an obstructive radiologist, this has to be addressed (E). As you are unlikely to know the registrar and work in a different department, you should attempt to escalate the issue up your own hierarchy first (B). If this is unsuccessful and you are still having difficulty, you could approach a senior doctor within the radiology department (e.g. the Clinical Director) (D). However, this would be a bold step and is best done with the support of your Clinical or Educational Supervisor. Opening a dialogue at the radiology meeting (C) could be helpful if there are specific structural issues which you are making a case to improve. However, it would be inappropriate to raise concerns about a specific colleague at this forum and anything less would be ineffective. The Mess President is unlikely to contribute very much to a meeting with the obstructive registrar (A).

16. C, E, F

It is important for medical professionals to ensure their own personal health and well-being. In this scenario, your SHO has revealed a serious psychological symptom which needs to be addressed (B). This might be alleviated through some form of counselling (D) or with antidepressants (G), although she initially requires a full medical assessment by an independent and objective healthcare professional (E). Professionally, she may benefit from the advice and support of her Educational Supervisor who has responsibility for her pastoral care (F). It is also reasonable to offer your own time and attention if she feels that she can speak freely to you (C), but you should avoid false reassurances (A).

17. B, C, D

All health professionals have a duty to protect their patients, and we should always be aware of the potential risk to children and vulnerable adults. Nevertheless, we also have a duty to respect our colleagues, and in this scenario it would be inappropriate to raise a serious concern in front of an unnecessary audience (E) without first establishing more information (C) and speaking to the SHO privately (D). It may then be appropriate to share your concerns with your consultant (B), who might involve more senior colleagues if necessary (A) (F). Informing the patient's family before establishing all the facts is premature and risks unnecessarily compromising the patient's trust if unfounded. If a serious assault has occurred, this would be managed by much more senior doctors (G). However, no doctor should conspire to silence patients and therefore should avoid telling patients what they can and cannot say (H).

18. B, C, D

Your Educational Supervisor has responsibility for providing appropriate supervision. This includes finding time for regular meetings. The scenario suggests that you have made substantial efforts to make alternative arrangements, without any meaningful success (H). You might wish to try again to arrange a more effective meeting (C); otherwise it appears reasonable to initiate the process of finding a suitable replacement (D) (G). It would be irresponsible to sign an educational (or any other) agreement without being aware of its contents (A) (B). It is not your responsibility to ask another consultant to take over the role of Educational Supervisor (E), and involving the deanery would not be a measured response at this stage (F).

19. A, B, E, D, C

As a junior trainee, your control over a project may not always correlate with your efforts. This should not preclude you from striving for fairness. In this instance, your hard work might be compensated with the chance to present some of your work (A). It might be unreasonable to ask the registrar to prepare a presentation for you the following week, but collaborating on further presentations might be helpful (B). However, there is value in preparing a presentation which should be recognized (E), and doing nothing would be a more measured response than refusing to share your slides (D) or involving your consultant (C).

20. **B, C, D, A, E**

Doctors should not treat themselves and taking medication from a drug cupboard is likely to contravene Trust policy. Ideally, the registrar should book in to the Emergency Department if necessary to obtain a prescription drug (B). Alternatively, you could prescribe omeprazole if you are willing to accept responsibility for the prescription (C). However, you should recall that symptoms of heartburn might indicate more serious pathology. You should raise any concerns about inappropriate administration of prescription drugs, ideally with those involved (D), before escalating them further (A). Doing nothing is, as usual, an unacceptable response (E).

21. **C, B, E, A, D**

GMC guidance states that all doctors must declare any caution or criminal conviction received anywhere in the world (D). Your professional relationship is more likely to be preserved by speaking to Peter and encouraging him to inform the GMC himself (C), or via his Educational Supervisor (B), before you personally declare it (A). Speaking to James will not change the situation as any caution which is received must be declared irrespective of the nature of the criminal offence (E).

22. **A, C, E, D, B**

It is not obvious from this scenario that there is any immediate danger to patients, although cannulation is a fundamental skill for any junior doctor and your colleague must learn to master it quickly. Hence, if it is possible to train him to cannulate effectively yourself, with minimal disruption to your duties, this should be attempted (A). It is better to encourage your colleague to seek senior support (C) rather than impose it upon him (E). The problem is not one which could be resolved immediately, and does not warrant fast-bleeping your consultant (D). The problem should not be ignored (B).

23. **D, E, C, B, A**

This is a very challenging situation which depends on a number of factors, particularly how confident you are that a mistake has been made and whether this can be reversed if correctly identified intraoperatively. This is an issue of patient safety and you have a duty to raise concerns immediately (D); not raising the issue is professionally unacceptable (A). It is less desirable to have to contact the consultant yourself without the registrar's agreement, but this may be necessary (E).

Raising the issue after the procedure may reduce the chance of reversing any error (C). However, involving the anaesthetist is also unhelpful as they are unlikely to have seen what happened or be willing to become involved in your disagreement (B).

24. A, C, F

Although Jill probably brings a wealth of knowledge and experience to the team, it is also important to foster a positive environment in which all members of the team are respected. It may not immediately impact on patient care but, indirectly, poor working relationships are likely to lead to less efficient care in the long term and so the issue should be addressed (A) (H). Effective work within a multi-disciplinary team requires mutual respect, rather than trying to establish dominance or accepting subordination (B) (D) (E). Nevertheless, your position of equal worth within the team may be reiterated by adopting a more confident approach (C). Asking the nursing staff whether they find Jill difficult to work is a leading question, implies fault, and is unlikely to gain you favour with her colleagues (G). In any challenging scenario, it is rarely incorrect to approach a senior colleague for advice (F).

25. D, A, B, C, E

Your response to Annabelle's request must balance exercise of your clinical judgement with maintaining an effective working relationship. The latter would not be achieved by insisting on your decision without further explanation (B) (A). Given Annabelle's confidence in her judgement and the fact that she has not accepted your initial explanation, it may be sensible (and diplomatic) to discuss her concerns with a senior colleague at a convenient time (D). However, if they are not clinically indicated, it would not be appropriate to commence anti-hypertensives. Prescribing them initially but stopping them later on (C) would be deceptive and confusing for the patient. You should certainly not suggest that a drug is administered without a prescription (E).

26. E, A, C, B, D

You should respect the ability of colleagues to deliver their own specialist services and manage their workload. However, this must be balanced with a duty to advocate for your patient.

In this case, you should speak to the psychologist to determine whether they are happy with their current input (E). They might agree or give reasons as to why so little time is being spent with Vera (e.g. volume of patients requiring attention or staffing pressures). You might want to discuss with other multi-disciplinary team members in case a consensus emerges as to how best Vera can be supported (A). You could certainly accept the psychologist's plan (they are likely to know best), but any concerns you have are best raised (C). Although patients can sometimes attend multi-disciplinary team meetings, this is unusual and probably inappropriate as other patients are usually discussed as well (B). It is not your place to instruct the psychologist as to the time they should spend and this is unlikely to be well received (D).

27. D, A, C, E, B

The most appropriate person arriving at a cardiac arrest should assume the role of team leader. In most cases, this will be the most senior doctor present, even if that person is an FY1. A cardiac arrest should be managed according to established protocols. However, whether the arrest is successful depends in part on how well it is led and whether each team member's skills are optimally utilized.

In this case, you should ask the medical student to find a crash trolley while you begin chest compressions (D). The nurse is likely to be exhausted at this point and the student should know what a crash trolley looks like. The student could be asked to continue chest compressions (A), but this assumes that they are confident and have good technique. Similarly, the domestic assistant might leave in search of a crash trolley (C) without knowing what they are looking for. Although you can certainly gain information from the nurse in attendance, you should assume responsibility for the arrest (E), particularly if the nurse is occupied doing compressions. It would be inappropriate to ask a medical student to lead the arrest regardless of how confident or competent you thought they were (B).

28. B, D, A, C, E

The pharmacist's request appears unnecessary and at best non-urgent. Other healthcare professionals should not generally attempt to prioritize your work as no one else can really understand the pressures on you at any one time. However, as the pharmacist is concerned, you should offer to raise the issue with a senior at a convenient time (B). Alternatively, a conciliatory approach might be to offer to complete the task later on (D). However, this risks being unable to do so because of other commitments and disappointing the pharmacist. The pharmacist is unlikely to call your consultant to demand completion of a non-urgent task. However, challenging her to do so (A) would be an unhelpful response and might embroil your consultant unnecessarily in the dispute. Nevertheless this is better than neglecting more important tasks (e.g. reviewing your patients so that the consultant can make better plans on his ward round) to keep the pharmacist happy (C). Clearly, the on-call team has more urgent demands on its time than amending prescriptions, and this would not be an appropriate task to hand over (E).

29. E, B, D, C, A

You must balance your workload (including answering your bleep) against the risk of dissuading the nurse from bleeping doctors in future. You should first listen to the nurse so that she can be satisfied that you have all the details and to ensure that this really is another inappropriate bleep (E). She may not be aware of the skeleton medical team available out of hours, and this might be a valuable education point (B). You could accept the task (D) but this risks causing you to neglect other responsibilities and does nothing to reduce inappropriate bleeping in future. Senior nurses sometimes triage bleeps to reduce pressure on the medical team out of hours. However, if this is not already local policy, you risk antagonizing the ward staff by suggesting it (C) at this point. You should certainly not stop the nurse from telephoning again, as next time it might be a genuine emergency (A).

30. C, D, A, B, E

The radiologist must also be satisfied than an investigation is indicated before agreeing that it should take place. This can lead to difficulties as the most junior person on the team (who probably has the least understanding of why the scan is necessary) is expected to communicate with the radiology consultant.

In this case, you should return to your consultant (C). He might clarify his particular reason for needing an ultrasound scan or think of a different approach to the same problem. Speaking with the radiologist in person might help (D) but only if you are armed with additional information— simply harrassing them to accept your request is unlikely to succeed. It is bad form to speak to another consultant as a way of skirting a decision made by their colleague (A). Similarly, a confrontational approach is unlikely to succeed and is best left to your own seniors if necessary (B). Although the radiologist has refused the request, this must be brought to the attention of your seniors in case they need to intervene or alter their management accordingly (E).

31. B, E, G

Although a discharge summary is clinically non-urgent, the patient has already been put to some inconvenience waiting for it to be completed. The regular team should have anticipated a weekend discharge and completed the summary.

You should certainly apologize for the delay so that it is clear that the wait was necessary (B). You could complete the discharge summary from the notes to the best of your ability but ask the regular team to make arrangements for follow-up (E). This will prevent the patient from having to attend an appointment unnecessarily or being prematurely discharged from surgical care. Although asking the patient to contact the team (C) might challenge his faith in the system, it is an honest approach and adds another layer of reassurance that follow-up will take place.

As the discharge summary is clinically non-urgent, you should not interrupt the surgical registrar in theatre (A). Neither the medical registrar (G) nor the GP (F) should be expected to determine the appropriateness of surgical follow-up. A routine follow-up appointment (D) might ensure further contact with the surgical team but may unnecessarily waste everyone's time.

The patient should not be asked to self-discharge (H) as the only reason for him to remain in hospital is administrative.

32. B, C, D

Booking annual leave in advance can be difficult as rotas are not published and you might not be currently based at the relevant hospital. However, this should not be an impenetrable barrier and you are entitled to make annual leave requests in advance (F) (G). You should aim to let all appropriate people at the hospital know your intention so that workforce arrangements can be made. These people are likely to include (at a minimum) your new Clinical Supervisor (C) and the rota coordinator (D). Once the rota is published, you will be responsible for arranging to swap any on-call shifts (B).

Your current Clinical Supervisor is unlikely to have very much influence, particularly if your leave request involves a different hospital (H). A formal letter of complaint (A) is unlikely to have much impact, might antagonize future colleagues, and will not change the annual leave policy. It is not your responsibility to arrange locum cover for any shifts that you might miss (E).

33. **A, B, E, C, D**

The two most important qualities of an FY1 doctor are effective communication skills and an ability to prioritize. Informing the phlebotomy team about your dilemma early on increases the likelihood of them being able to help (A). This would permit you to see the outpatient who has been waiting for some time and therefore should be prioritized (B). You could certainly ask another FY1 for assistance if this does not distract them from their own commitments (E).

It would be inappropriate, and unlikely to foster positive working relationships, if you were to hand over your tasks to the ward team (C). However, you might enlist the help of nurses who are able to take blood if they are available to do so. Although it is worth taking a few minutes to prioritize tasks, taking a coffee break at this point (D) would waste time and risk leaving a patient waiting unnecessarily in the outpatient department.

34. **B, C, E**

Your patient may benefit from all manner of services but you must balance this against the appropriateness of each referral.

The patient's GP (B) will provide long-term follow-up and will be able to access many different services of potential benefit to your patient. He may also require specialist drug and alcohol input which can be provided by an appropriately qualified person (C). A social worker (E) could also help assess the patient's need for additional services.

The Ward Sister is not likely to expect continued involvement with this man unless he becomes an inpatient again (A). Similarly, there is no reason to think that he would benefit substantially from housing services (D), the Citizen's Advice Bureau (F), a psychologist (G), or the transplant service (H). These may become necessary in future, which is all the more reason to ensure that he remains engaged with key people such as his GP and social services.

35. **A, B, D, C, E**

Handover is not only important between shifts, but it is also necessary when moving jobs. You should endeavour to leave all routine tasks completed and a clear set of instructions for your successor.

If there are ways of improving the induction process, you should let an appropriate person (e.g. your Clinical Supervisor) know (A). You should also leave a detailed note for your successor which contains post-specific advice, such as schedules, useful bleep numbers, and hard-learned tips (B). You might also want to leave contact details (D) in case anything is unclear, particularly about where things have been left or the patients whom you looked after. It would usually be excessive to take time off to support your successor. This would defeat the purpose of annual leave (rest and recuperation!) and disrupt your new team which would have to cope without its FY1 in the first week (C).

You have a duty to make improvements when this is within your sphere of influence. The Foundation Programme induction will cover many areas, but cannot provide the post-specific advice which is likely to be most useful to your successor (E).

36. B, A, C, D, E

Although people will have different priorities, a minimum standard of professional behaviour is expected of all doctors. This is usually enforced informally.

In this case, the transgression is relatively minor and so requires a measured approach. You should first ask the SHO whether there is a problem (B), as this will bring the issue to his attention. There may actually be a problem (e.g. an emergency at home) and it might be appropriate for him to leave the ward round. You should also let him know that others have noticed so that he is aware of the impact of his behaviour (A). Asking the SHO to put his phone away (C) might not be received very well and is unlikely to have the desired effect. The remaining options, i.e. informing the consultant (D) and initiating a 'politeness code' (E), would not be measured responses to the situation described.

37. E, D, C, B, A

In any difficult situation involving colleagues, it is important to establish the facts early on (E). You might be willing to help out your SHO if there is a temporary problem with childcare but she will be working normal hours in the near future.

If it is likely to become a long-term problem, it would be necessary to confront the SHO directly. You must make it clear that you are unwilling to accept the current arrangement (D) which risks patient safety and your own well-being. If the matter cannot be resolved through discussion, it must be escalated to your consultant (C). Although time might be made up elsewhere, working through lunch is not an optimal long-term strategy and should not be imposed on the SHO (B). Asking her to cover your early mornings (A) is the least safe option as it leaves only one doctor on site for 1.5 hours every day.

38. **B, E, G**

The immediate goal should be to de-escalate what could become an inflammatory situation if an argument was to develop. Your best move would be to steer the ward round back to its original business of reviewing patients (B). However, you should also let the registrar know afterwards that his behaviour raised concerns (E). If this is unsuccessful, the matter should be raised with your consultant (G).

You should avoid becoming embroiled in controversial discussions when these are likely to cause offence in the workplace. This includes agreeing (D) or disagreeing (C) with the registrar.

It would be an overreaction to leave the ward round (F) or apologize on your registrar's behalf (A), although he might wish to approach the patient after you have brought the issue to his attention. Similarly, you should not usually solicit complaints from patients about colleagues (H).

39. **E, B, A, C, D**

Dishonest removal of hospital equipment constitutes theft with its attendant legal and professional consequences. You should insist tghat your colleague returns any property which has been removed (E) and that you will take the matter further if he continues to take items without permission (B).

You might wish to let the theatre manager know that property is going missing (A) so that items can be appropriately secured and warnings distributed to staff.

The only justification for not reporting your colleague outright (C) is that he might not have fully considered the consequences of this action. If he had stolen something more obvious (e.g. a hospital PC), you would clearly have to involve the hospital authorities early on.

However, you should not accept the situation as it currently stands (D). Although a surgical registrar could argue that the Trust should make reasonable allowances for practice, this is less convincing for an FY1. Instead, he is forcing his employer to subsidize his further professional education without their agreement.

40. **C, E, F**

Attending a set number of teaching sessions is a mandatory requirement for completion of FY1. If you identify difficulties attending sessions, these must be raised early on so that you do not find yourself in difficulty towards the end of the year.

You could certainly speak with the SHO to emphasize the importance of sufficient cover so that you can attend teaching (E). However, the issue should be escalated swiftly if it persists. Your Clinical Supervisor (C) is a good place to start, followed by your Educational Supervisor if issues are still not resolved. It would also be polite to inform the teaching coordinator as well by way of apology for not arriving (F).

You should not leave the clinic without cover, particularly if you doubt that your SHO will arrive on time (A). Similarly, you should not delegate to another healthcare professional (G) unless this has been agreed locally. The secretaries are unlikely to be able to manipulate the clinic volume without impacting on the elective operating list (H). Involving a senior doctor for the simple task of reminding your SHO is unlikely to be received well (B). Asking a colleague to sign you in to teaching casts doubt on both your own and your colleague's probity (D).

Section 3

Practice test

Chapter 14

Practice test

This chapter presents a practice test with a mix of question types (e.g. multiple choice or ranking), content (e.g. domain tested), and styles (e.g. patient, colleague, or personal). It includes 30 questions and broadly reflects the type of questions likely to be asked in the SJT (p. 11). To make the most of this test, you should complete it in one sitting within an hour before checking your answers (p. 214).

When checking your answers to ranking questions, remember that credit is still given for 'near misses' and so there is no need to hit the 'correct' sequence every time (p. 9).

The practice test answers are not accompanied by detailed explanations. For this reason, it would be preferable to complete all the questions in Section 2 (pp. 27–196) before attempting the test.

To replicate the SJT as closely as possible, you should ideally complete these questions within an hour under formal examination conditions. Once you have attempted all the questions, turn to p. 214 to check your answers. It is difficult to interpret your final score as your rank will depend entirely on how well your colleagues (and every other medical student in the country) fare.

If you are organized, you could arrange a study group to work through this book and/or complete the practice test. Marking your answers as a group will give some indication as to your performance relative to others. It will also provide an opportunity to discuss the various options (including disagreement with our answers) and so gain a deeper understanding of the issues tested by the SJT.

QUESTIONS

1. You are working as an FY1 in the Medical Assessment Unit, seeing Marcin who is a 35-year-old Polish man with very limited English language skills.

Rank in order the following actions in response to this situation
(1 = Most appropriate; 5 = Least appropriate)

A Attempt a brief history using hand gestures and diagrams.

B Try to contact a member of Marcin's family to act as an interpreter over the phone.

C Do not attempt a history without a translator present.

D Skip the history, and focus your management on the examination and investigations.

E Extrapolate a history based on the limited findings of the ambulance crew on their initial assessment sheet.

2. During a GP rotation you see Carl, who would like to know the results of a colonoscopy and CT scan after a joint MDT meeting. He missed his last appointment, but has been told that the GP should have access to the report. The results identify a disseminated colorectal malignancy, although no treatment plan has yet been decided upon.

Rank in order the following actions in response to this situation
(1 = Most appropriate; 5 = Least appropriate)

A Establish what the patient understands about his diagnosis first.

B Refer him back to the gastroenterologist who performed the colonoscopy.

C Contact the nurse specialist and ask her to telephone the patient as soon as possible.

D Explain the very poor outcome associated with cancers like the one Carl has.

E Ask the patient to come back and see you in the afternoon, as you will need to speak to his hospital doctors first.

3. During a busy urology ward round with your consultant, the nurse mentions that Frank, who is recovering from a transurethral resection of prostate, has admitted to feeling low over the last few months.

Choose the THREE most appropriate actions to take in this situation

A Ask the consultant to speak to Frank about his low mood.

B Speak to Frank after the ward round.

C Ask Frank if he is low enough for antidepressants.

D Break away from the ward round to discuss the matter with Frank.

E Ask the nurse to keep any additional patient information until the end of the ward round to avoid future interruptions.

F Inform your seniors after the ward round, if a referral needs to be made.

G Tell the patient to speak to someone about his low mood.

H Inform the on-call psychiatrist.

4. You are asked to see Jerry, a 55-year-old man who has recently undergone a colonic resection with defunctioning colostomy. He wishes to make a complaint against the operating consultant as he feels that he was not adequately informed about the impact of his stoma.

Rank in order the following actions in response to this situation
(1 = Most appropriate; 5 = Least appropriate)

A Inform the patient that you will relay his concerns to the consultant.

B Apologize on the consultant's behalf.

C Establish the difficulties that Jerry has been having with the stoma.

D Defend the consultant by explaining that the formation of a stoma was documented on the consent form.

E Inform the patient of the complaints procedure and how he might go about registering a complaint.

5. Your registrar shouts at a medical student in front of a patient. The medical student comes to find you afterwards in tears and is uncertain how to react to this treatment.

Rank in order the following actions in response to this situation
(1 = Most appropriate; 5 = Least appropriate)

A Suggest that the student report the registrar to an appropriate person within the medical school.

B Bleep your registrar and ask him to return to the ward and apologize to the medical student.

C Apologize on behalf of the registrar, and ask the student not to say anything to anyone else.

D Suggest that the student talk to the firm consultant about the episode.

E Tell the student that they would be less likely to provoke a negative response if their knowledge base was better.

6. You are a lone FY1 seeing a postoperative patient with atrial fibrillation and a heart rate of 160 bpm. Before you finish your assessment, the patient starts to mumble incoherently and will not follow commands or open his eyes.

Choose the THREE most appropriate actions to take in this situation

A Ensure that the patient has a valid Not For Rescusitation order in case they suffer cardiac arrest.

B Accept that 160 bpm might be normal for this patient.

C Shout for help.

D Ask the nursing staff to put out a peri-arrest call.

E Ensure that you have good intravenous access and give a fluid challenge.

F Ask the patient's family to attend as their relative is probably dying.

G Start chest compressions.

H Ensure that you have adequate airway adjuncts to hand.

7. Your FY1 colleague takes a copy of the operating list home every evening to prepare for the following day in theatre.

Rank in order the following actions in response to this situation
(1 = Most appropriate; 5 = Least appropriate)

A Suggest that your colleague makes a simple list of operations to take home.

B Take your own list home so that you can prepare for the theatre list as well.

C Suggest that it is unfair he is 'getting ahead'.

D Speak to the consultant about your colleague's behaviour.

E Inform your colleague that he should not be taking home any list containing confidential patient information.

8. The registrar asks you to teach two medical students who have only just begun their training. You have a long list of jobs to complete and your SHO has just called in sick.

Rank in order the following actions in response to this situation
(1 = Most appropriate; 5 = Least appropriate)

A Tell the registrar that you are too busy to look after students.

B Allow the students to shadow you for half an hour, and then ask them to leave.

C Ask the students to attempt to take blood from a few of the patients in exchange for some teaching.

D Allow the students to shadow you completing your routine jobs, before sending them to take a history from a few patients.

E Postpone your ward jobs in order to teach the students for an hour.

9. Your registrar informs you that there is a peritonitic patient intubated on the intensive therapy unit (ITU), waiting to be transferred back to theatre. You have never felt a genuine 'surgical abdomen' before, and are keen to utilize this opportunity.

Choose the THREE most appropriate actions to take in this situation

A Do not examine the patient as you have not obtained consent.

B Send a text message to another FY1 to suggest that he examines the patient as well.

C Use this opportunity to read up about causes of 'surgical abdomen'.

D Examine the patient as this is a valuable learning opportunity.

E Try to contact the patient's next of kin to ask if you can examine the patient.

F Complete your routine ward tasks before going to see the patient.

G Introduce yourself to the ITU consultant and ask if you can examine the patient.

H Go and see the patient but do not examine their abdomen.

10. You are a new FY1 in surgery, and have been asked to see a patient in urinary retention who requires a catheter. You have only ever performed catheterization on a model and are not feeling particularly confident.

Rank in order the following actions in response to this situation
(1 = Most appropriate; 5 = Least appropriate)

A Attempt the procedure after talking to the patient, and then ask for help if unsuccessful.

B Call the registrar and ask them to supervise your first catheterization.

C Attempt the procedure without warning the patient about your inexperience.

D Ask another FY1 who is more confident with procedures to help.

E Wait until the end of your shift and then hand the job over to the night team.

11. You are driving home from your evening on call when you remember a chest X-ray which needed to be reviewed for a patient with a newly inserted chest drain. You forgot to hand it over to your colleague who was taking over.

Rank in order the following actions in response to this situation
(1 = Most appropriate; 5 = Least appropriate)

A Put the issue out of your mind—it's important to 'turn off' after work.

B Make a note to check the result first thing in the morning before the ward round.

C Drive back to the hospital to check the X-ray yourself.

D Contact the on-call doctor through the switchboard and ask them to check the X-ray.

E Reflect about the factors which might have led to forgetting the X-ray.

12. You are working on call covering the medical wards. The registrar asks you to place a chest drain in a patient with a confirmed empyema who is becoming increasingly breathless. As a respiratory FY1 you have seen many chest tubes being inserted, but have yet to place one. The registrar is very busy and will not be able to help.

Choose the THREE most appropriate actions to take in this situation

A Call the registrar and explain that you cannot safely perform the procedure alone but would be grateful if he could supervise you.

B Call the registrar back to say that you are unwilling to do as he asks.

C Use the *Oxford Handbook for the Foundation Programme* to guide your attempt at independently inserting the chest drain.

D Begin to insert the chest drain and contact the on-call registrar if you encounter difficulties.

E Contact your Educational Supervisor at the first possible opportunity to discuss the appropriateness of this request.

F Contact another senior colleague if the on-call registrar does not answer or offers no further support.

G Set up the equipment and explain the procedure to the patient.

H Remind the registrar of the chest drain again in a couple of hours when he is less busy.

13. You are looking after Sally who has become increasingly unwell due to heart failure, despite maximal diuretic therapy. Both you and your registrar believe that Sally would benefit from inotrope therapy on ITU. The patient's son and the nursing staff feel that aggressive escalation of treatment would not benefit Sally.

Rank in order the following actions in response to this situation
(1 = Most appropriate; 5 = Least appropriate)

A Refer Sally to ITU as you are ultimately responsible for the patient.

B Read through the medical notes, and try to understand why the family and nursing staff might not want to escalate treatment.

C Tell the patient's brother and nursing staff to think carefully about the options and that you will do as they want if all members agree.

D Document your discussion with the family and stop all active treatment in order to ameliorate the patient's suffering.

E Contact a senior doctor to ask them to make a decision.

14. You are just starting your shift as the evening on-call medical FY1 and have been handed over along list of jobs as well as answering bleeps from nursing staff. You need to prioritize tasks.

Rank in order the following actions in response to this situation
(1 = Most appropriate; 5 = Least appropriate)

A An upset patient who wants to discuss her forthcoming endoscopy on the next day.

B An 80-year-old man who has had a fall and hit his head, but appears lucid.

C A 70-year-old with a past history of myocardial infarction who has just become unresponsive.

D A 50-year-old man after an elective herniotomy who is still awaiting prescription laxatives and pain killers before he can be discharged.

E A 30-year-old man with renal colic requiring analgesia review for '10/10' pain.

15. You are working as the orthopaedic FY1, when you are called by the orthopaedic registrar on your mobile about a patient who will be arriving on the private ward. He asks you to clerk, cannulate, and initiate intravenous fluids, as the patient will be undergoing elective surgery the following morning.

*Rank in order the following actions in response to this situation
(1 = Most appropriate; 5 = Least appropriate)*

A Prioritise the preoperative clerking and fluid administration alongside your other tasks.

B Contact a responsible person (e.g. duty manager) to ask about the appropriateness of doing jobs on the private ward.

C Suggest that the registrar comes in to complete the clerking if he has agreed to see the consultant's private patient.

D Help if possible, but inform the registrar that this is not a long-term solution for managing private patients.

E Agree to complete the tasks for a reasonable fee.

16. A 40-year-old patient is admitted for an elective procedure on your surgery ward. After reading an article in a newspaper about statins, he tells you he would like them to be prescribed. He is at low risk of cardiovascular disease.

*Rank in order the following actions in response to this situation
(1 = Most appropriate; 5 = Least appropriate)*

A Write a prescription for statins.

B Explain that the high cost of statins means they can only be prescribed to high-risk patients.

C Write to his GP asking them to discuss the patient's request.

D Inform the patient that he does not have a high enough risk of cardiac disease to gain sufficient benefit from the medication.

E Refer the problem to your consultant.

17. After a ward round, you are approached by one of the patients who says that they are 'scared' and no longer want a bronchoscopy the following day.

*Rank in order the following actions in response to this situation
(1 = Most appropriate; 5 = Least appropriate)*

A Discuss the patient's decision with the nursing staff.

B Explain the benefits of the procedure and insist that she receives it no matter what.

C Explore alternative investigations.

D Establish the patient's concerns.

E Consider whether the patient has capacity to refuse.

18. You are working in paediatrics, and have made two attempts at cannulating a 7-year-old with diabetic ketoacidosis. The mother is becoming quite frustrated and refuses any further attempts.

Choose the THREE most appropriate actions to take in this situation

A Tell the mother that the next attempt will be successful.

B Explain that you will ask a colleague to try if the next attempt fails.

C Encourage oral intake and clearly document that the parent refused cannulation.

D Stop the fluids and re-site the cannula if the patient deteriorates.

E Tell the mother that her daughter will probably die without intravenous fluids.

F Document the number of attempts at cannulation afterwards.

G Persist with cannulation attempts as the mother cannot refuse treatment on her child's behalf

H Explain carefully why a cannula is necessary.

19. You are an FY1 reviewing patients with your consultant. The consultant tells Doug, a 30-year-old man, that he has a staghorn calculus and must have an operation which will leave a nephrostomy. The consultant leaves once the consent form is signed but Doug looks as if he still has more questions.

Rank in order the following actions in response to this situation
(1 = Most appropriate; 5 = Least appropriate)

A Tell the patient that your consultant will come back later to answer questions.

B Explain that you will come back shortly in case he has any more questions.

C Insist that the consultant stays until he has answered his questions.

D Continue with reviewing patients with the consultant but see Doug later to answer any questions.

E Let your consultant continue reviewing other patients alone but remain behind to answer Doug's questions.

20. You have received several complaints from the nursing staff about Michael, who has learning difficulties and has been mobilizing unsafely around the ward. He has become increasingly challenging to manage.

Rank in order the following actions in response to this situation
(1 = Most appropriate; 5 = Least appropriate)

A Ask whether a 'special' nurse can be assigned for one-to-one care.

B Attempt to explain to Michael, as far as possible, that it is unsafe for him to move around the ward.

C Suggest distracting interventions.

D Prescribe 'as-required' (PRN) sedation.

E Prescribe sedation when Michael becomes particularly agitated and endangers himself or others.

21. Jessie was admitted under the gastroenterology team for chronic abdominal pain. Investigations have not yielded any findings, and your consultant believes that the patient should be discharged with follow-up from the pain team. The patient and her family do not believe she can go home with such severe pain.

Choose the THREE most appropriate actions to take in this situation

A Delete the patient from your list so that she can remain an inpatient for a few more days.

B Explore Jessie's concerns about going home.

C Promise that you will ensure that the pain team appointment is made within two weeks.

D Tell Jessie the bed is needed for more urgent cases.

E Carefully explain the nature of chronic abdominal pain.

F Ensure that the pain team is involved with discharge planning so that appropriate analgesia can be provided in the community.

G Prescribe 'as-required' (PRN) Oramorph until the patient is discharged.

H Tell Jessie that she needs to learn to accept the pain as it cannot be helped.

22. Six hours ago you prescribed intravenous antibiotics for a surgical patient for a suspected pelvic abscess. During your afternoon ward round you find that the antibiotics have still not been given by the nurse.

Rank in order the following actions in response to this situation
(1 = Most appropriate; 5 = Least appropriate)

A Contact the pharmacy and seek advice about how to prepare the infusion yourself.

B Inform the Ward Sister that the antibiotics have been dangerously delayed.

C Ensure that the nurse understands the importance of giving antibiotics promptly.

D Approach the nurse on her break and insist that she prepares the intravenous antibiotics immediately.

E Allow the nurse to complete her jobs without further instruction— she will administer the infusion when she has time.

23. Your SHO prescribes a large dose of gentamicin for a patient with severe renal failure. You notice this when rewriting the drug chart, thankfully before this renotoxic drug was administered. Your SHO thanks you for stopping the prescription in time.

Rank in order the following actions in response to this situation
(1 = Most appropriate; 5 = Least appropriate)

A Inform the hospital pharmacy.

B Record a critical incident form for a near miss.

C Inform your consultant at the next available opportunity.

D Do nothing further as the SHO simply forgot that caution is needed when prescribing gentamicin for patients with renal impairment.

E Note 'renal impairment' somewhere appropriate on the drug chart.

24. While eating lunch in the hospital canteen, you overhear a nurse describing a junior doctor as 'incompetent'. The doctor is readily identifiable but the nurse seems unaffected by the attention she is attracting from surrounding diners.

Rank in order the following actions in response to this situation
(1 = Most appropriate; 5 = Least appropriate)

A Speak to the nurse on the ward later on to explain that such comments in a public environment are unprofessional.

B Let the nurse know that she can be overheard by other diners.

C Speak to someone in the nursing hierarchy to reinforce the message about not publicly undermining colleagues.

D Let the junior doctor concerned know what was said about him.

E Do nothing as this is a public venue and the nurse is on her break.

25. An FY1 colleague who works on your ward consistently struggles to take blood from patients. The samples he has successfully obtained are usually haemolysed.

Rank in order the following actions in response to this situation
(1 = Most appropriate; 5 = Least appropriate)

A Ignore the problem as it is your colleague's concern.

B Email his Clinical Supervisor.

C Contact your consultant immediately to inform him of yourcolleague's difficulties.

D Help your colleague improve on the ward and by using a skills laboratory if there is one.

E Suggest that your colleague asks a senior for help.

26. You are finding it particularly difficult to work with your new SHO. She is condescending, undermines your management, and has often belittled you in front of senior colleagues.

Choose the THREE most appropriate actions to take in this situation

A Adopt a more subordinate position as her junior colleague.

B Ask your colleagues within the medical team whether they find your SHO difficult to work with.

C Do nothing, provided that her behaviour does not impact on clinical care.

D Ensure that your jobs are done well to avoid avoidable criticism.

E Remind the SHO about your relative inexperience in medicine.

F Speak to a senior colleague for advice.

G Discuss your feelings with the SHO.

H Try to challenge your SHO's clinical knowledge in an effort to impress her.

27. You have just started working on the care of the elderly ward. Despite your relative inexperience, you are certain that your consultant has recklessly discharged unwell patients many times over a four-week period. However, he is well regarded on the ward by patients and nurses. You have never heard another doctor complain about his practice.

Choose the THREE most appropriate actions to take in this situation

A Ask your consultant about specific discharges with which you are unhappy.

B Contact the GMC to raise your concerns.

C Record the events clearly on your medical blog.

D Do nothing as you are alone in thinking that the consultant's decisions are flawed.

E Do nothing as you have no real proof of poor practice.

F Discuss your concerns privately with another senior colleague.

G Contact your Educational Supervisor.

H Inform the Medical Director.

28. You are clerking a young child in the preoperative admissions clinic. You note that the parents are somewhat untidy, with dirty hands and clothes. You consider what to document this in the medical notes.

Rank in order the following actions in response to this situation
(1 = Most appropriate; 5 = Least appropriate)

A Complete your detailed entry into the notes once you have clerked everyone at the preoperative assessment clinic.

B Briefly summarize your clinical assessment.

C Document thhe impression that you have formed of the parent's suitability for raising the child.

D Document your detailed physical examination findings of the child.

E Write your notes once your senior colleagues agree with your findings.

29. You have just completed your assessment of a patient who is hypotensive and asked the nurses to administer intravenous fluids. You are bleeped by another ward to say that a patient is pyrexial. While you are taking this call, your crash bleep summons you to a third ward.

Rank in order the following actions in response to this situation
(1 = Most appropriate; 5 = Least appropriate)

A Many doctors carry crash bleeps and you should prioritize the patient you are currently treating.

B Attend the crash call but return later to document your assessment retrospectively.

C Document your current assessment of the patient who is hypotensive and then attend the crash call.

D See the febrile patient after the crash call and then return to document your approach to the hypotensive patient.

E Don't document anything as the unwell patients are a priority.

30. You are being shadowed by a medical student while on call. You receive three bleeps in quick succession: a respiratory patient looking increasingly unwell, blood cultures needed for a febrile patient, and a disgruntled relative wanting to complain about your consultant.

Choose the THREE most appropriate actions to take in this situation

A Ask the medical student to assess the respiratory patient, and you will review shortly afterwards.

B Review the respiratory patient with the medical student.

C Suggest that the student takes blood from the febrile patient.

D Review the respiratory patient alone.

E Do the blood cultures first in case the patient's fever subsides.

F Suggest that the student speaks to the disgruntled relative.

G Meet the relative by yourself on the ward.

H Speak to the relative together with a nurse in a side room.

ANSWERS

1. B, A, C, E, D
2. A, E, C, D, B
3. B, F, H
4. C, A, D, E, B
5. D, A, B, C, E
6. C, D, E
7. E, A, D, C, B
8. D, A, E, B, C
9. C, D, G
10. D, A, C, B, E
11. D, C, E, B, A
12. A, F, G
13. B, E, A, C, D
14. C, B, E, A, D
15. A, D, B, C, E
16. D, C, E, A, B
17. D, E, C, A, B
18. B, F, H
19. B, D, E, A, C
20. B, C, A, E, D
21. B, E, F
22. C, B, D, E, A
23. E, B, A, C, D
24. B, A, C, D, E
25. D, E, A, B, C
26. D, F, G
27. A, F, G
28. D, B, A, E, C
29. B, D, E, C, A
30. B, C, H

Index